Getting Ready for My Ear Tube Surgery

Ear Tubes Book for Kids – Preparation and Recovery

This book belongs to:

Written by Dr. Fei Zheng-Ward   Illustrated by Moch. Fajar Shobaru

Copyright © 2025 Fei Zheng-Ward

All rights reserved. Published by Fei Zheng-Ward, an imprint of FZWbooks. No part of this book may be copied, reproduced, recorded, transmitted, or stored by any means or in any form, electronic or mechanical, without obtaining prior written permission from the copyright owner.

Identifiers: ISBN 979-8-89318-061-9 (eBook)
                    ISBN 979-8-89318-062-6 (paperback)
                    ISBN 979-8-89318-066-4 (hardcover)

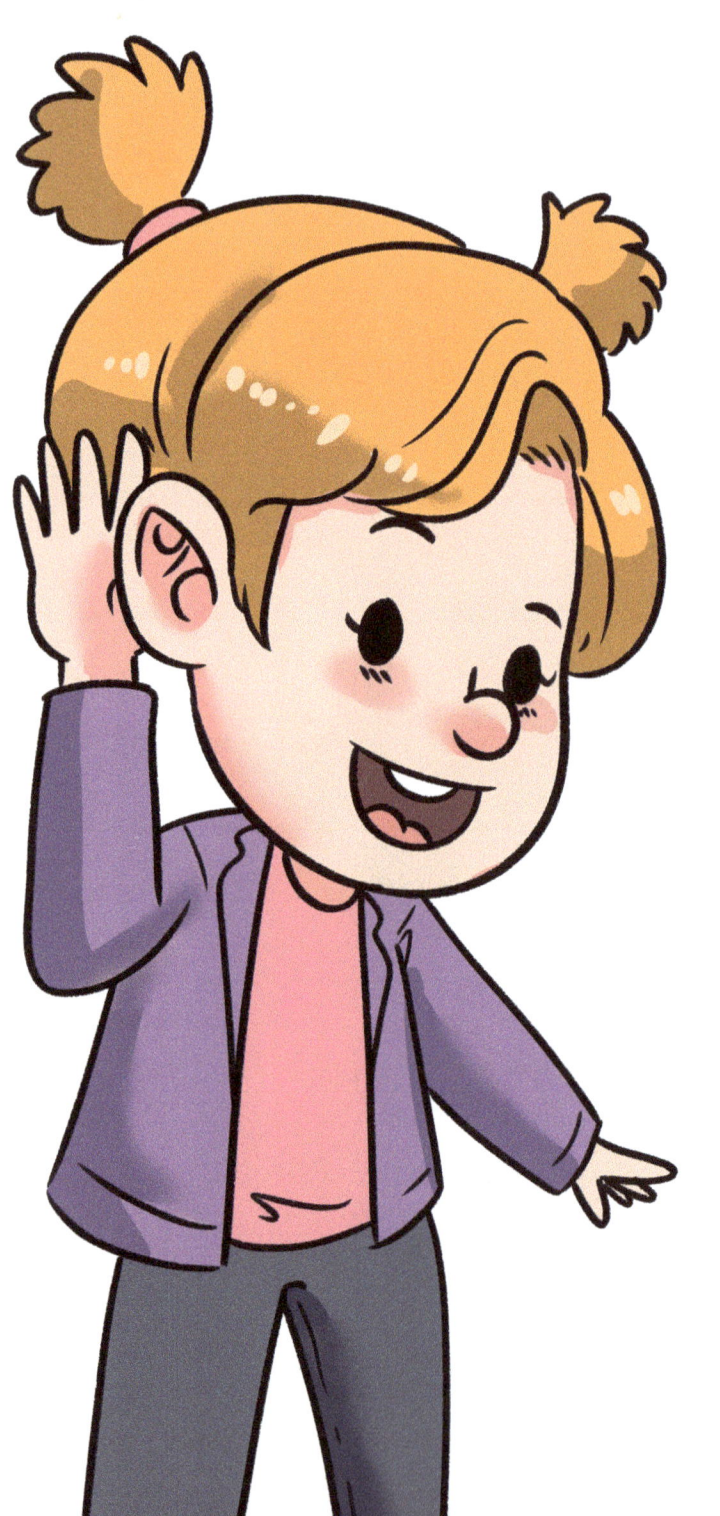

What's your favorite thing to listen to?

Music _____

A story _____

A funny joke _____

Whatever may be your favorite you need to hear well so you can learn and grow.

Did you know that each of your ears has three main parts?

They include the outer ear, the middle ear, and the inner ear.

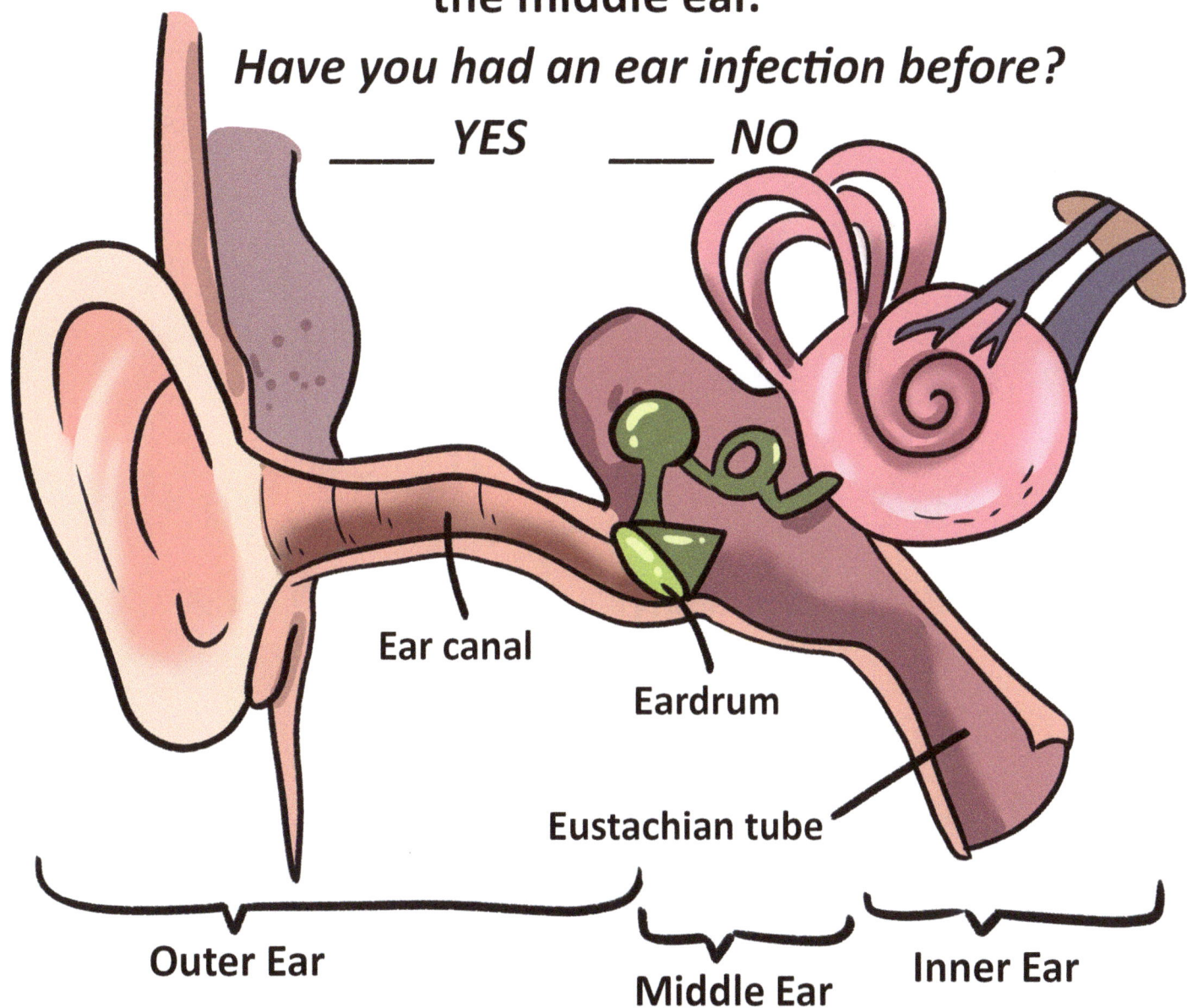

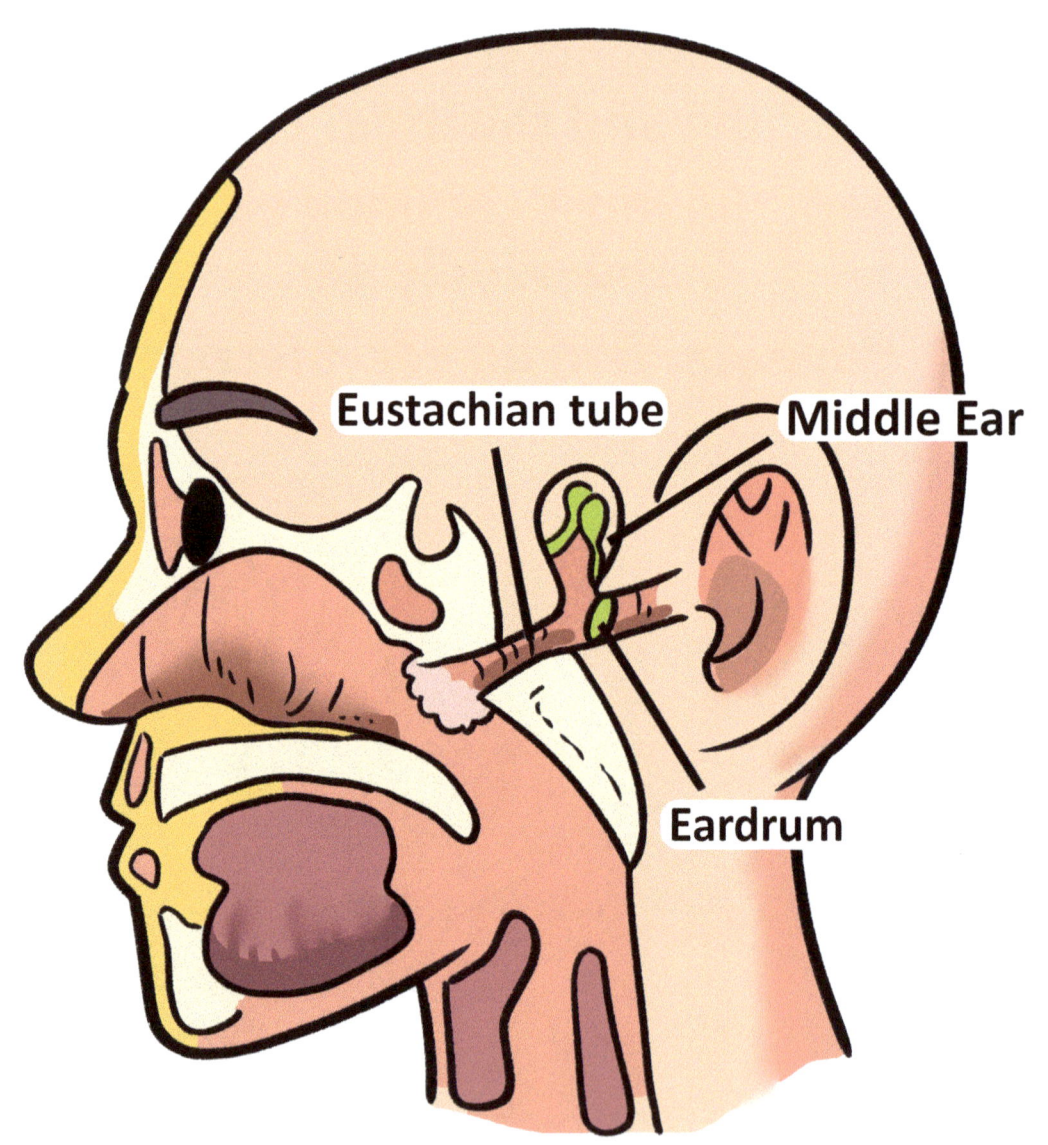

The Eustachian (yoo-stay-shuhn) tube connects the middle ear to the back of your nose and is normally closed. It opens occasionally to equalize pressure between your middle ear and the outside world.

When the tube opens, you may hear your ear pop.

Fun fact: Did you know you open your Eustachian tube when you open your mouth wide, yawn, gently blow your nose, suck on a lollipop, or swallow?

Pressure in your ear gives you the feeling that it is plugged up, full, or stuffy, and you cannot hear well.

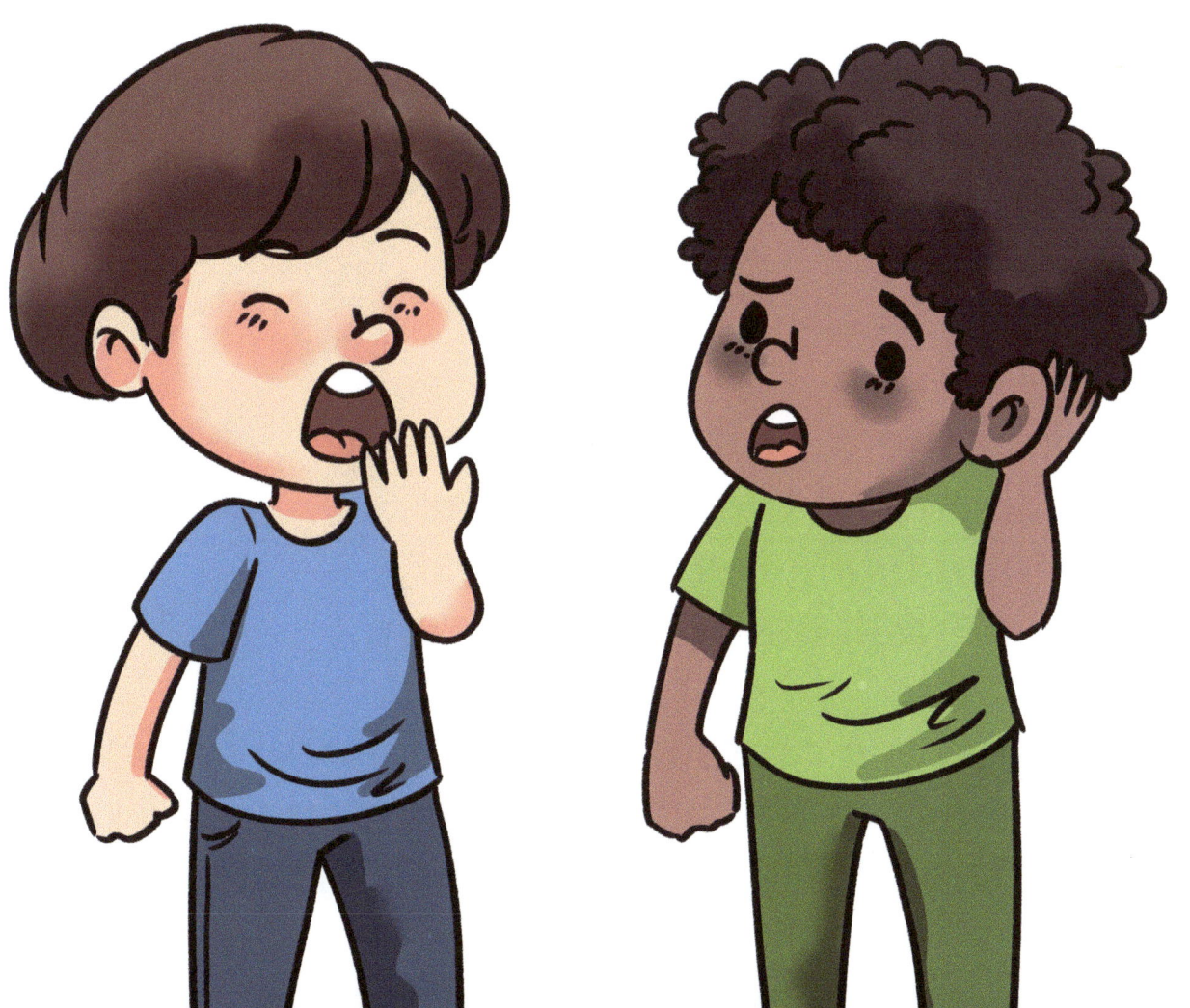

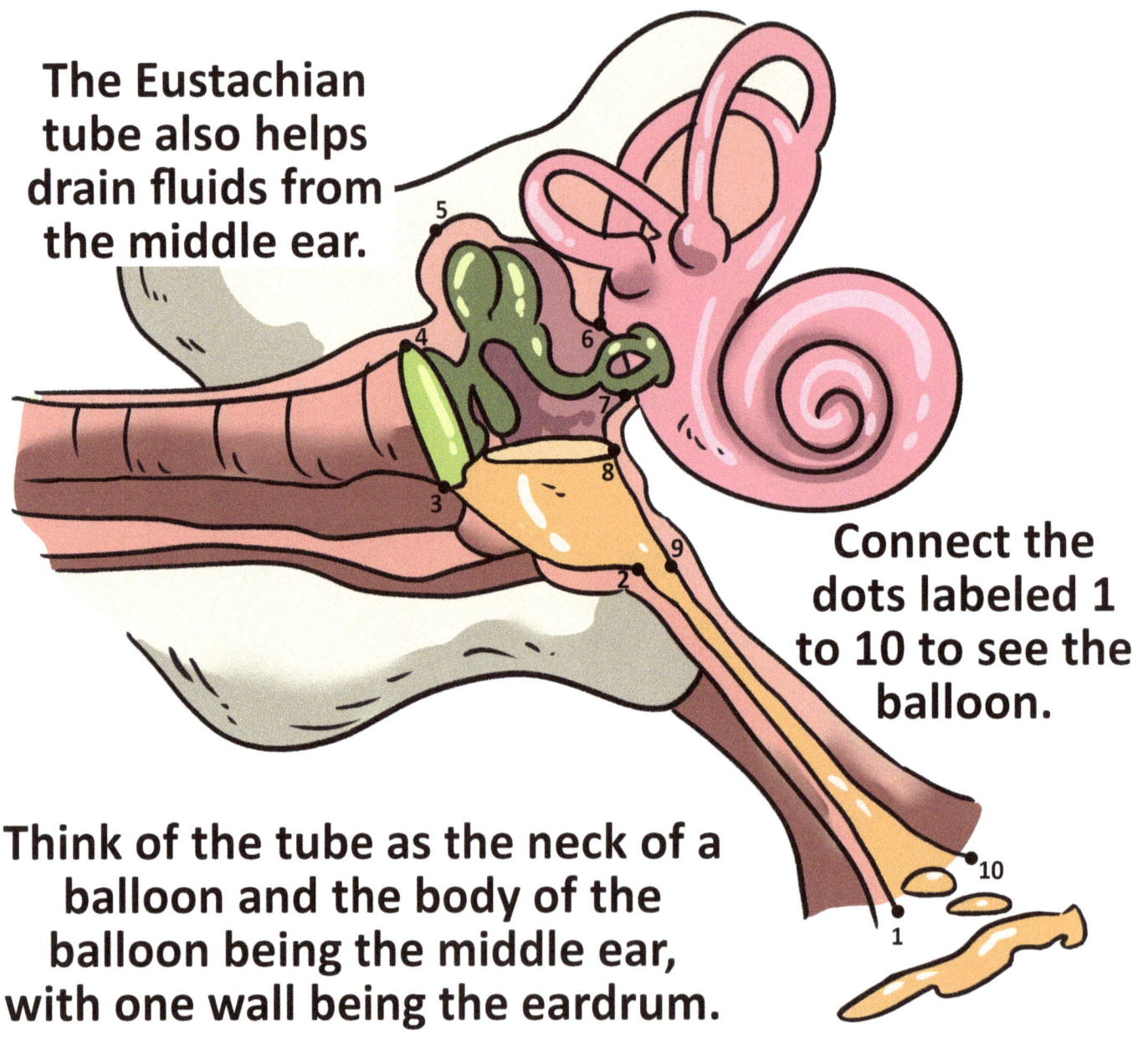

The Eustachian tube also helps drain fluids from the middle ear.

Connect the dots labeled 1 to 10 to see the balloon.

Think of the tube as the neck of a balloon and the body of the balloon being the middle ear, with one wall being the eardrum.

When the pressure in the balloon is too high, the neck of the balloon can open up to release the pressure. The opposite is also true.

The pressure inside your middle ear changes when you fly inside an airplane, go up or down a mountain, go diving, or are sick with a cold or have a sinus infection.

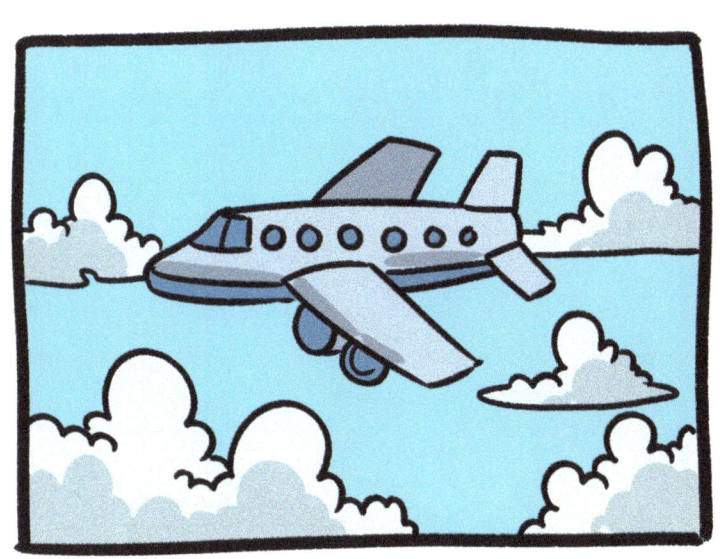
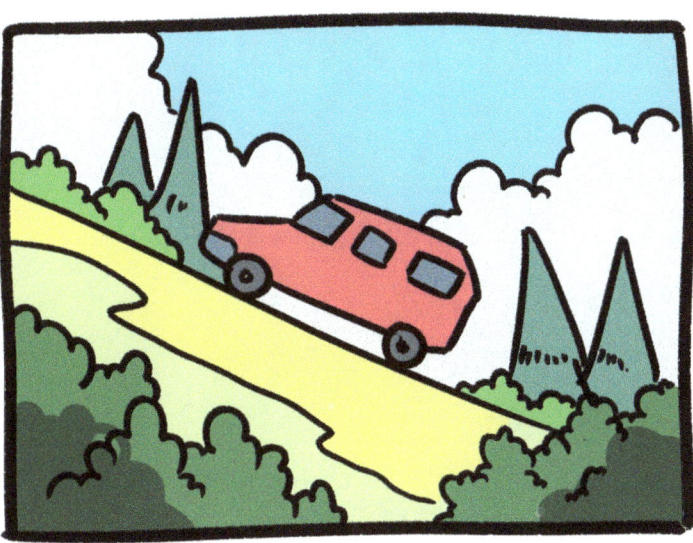
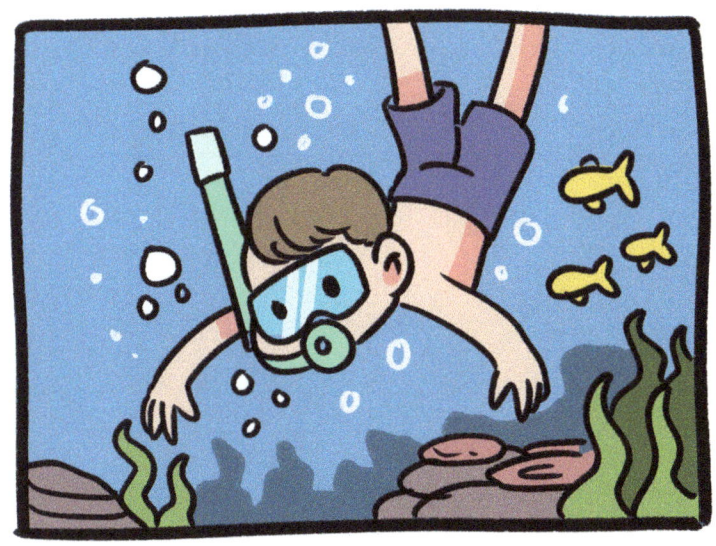
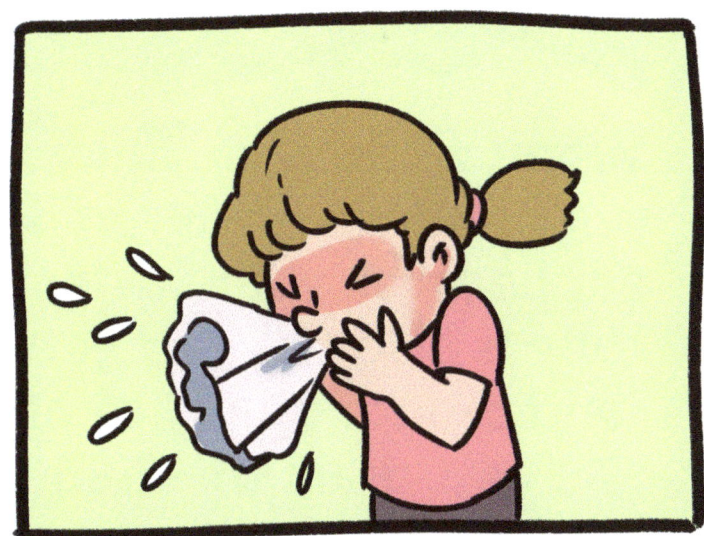

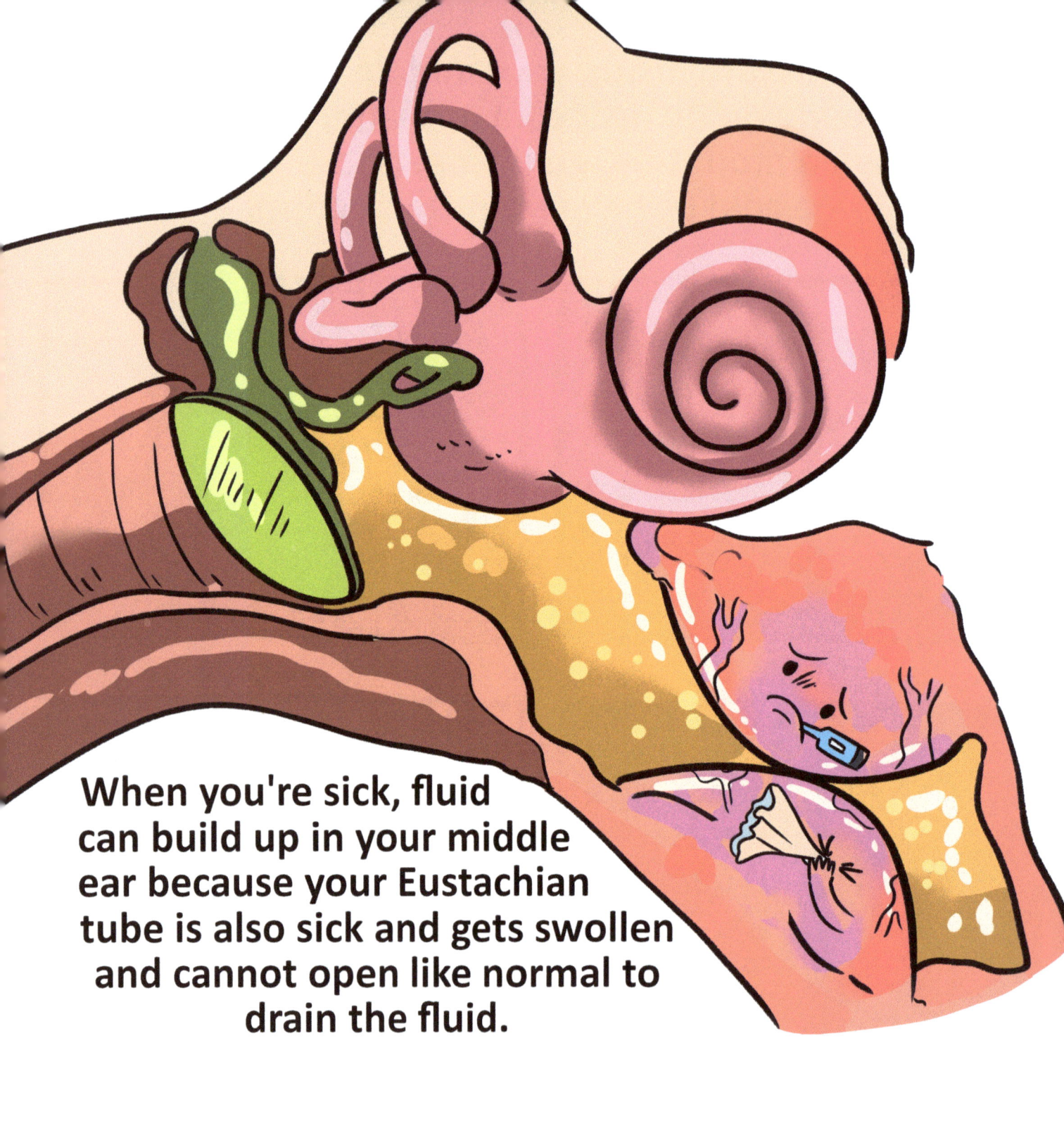

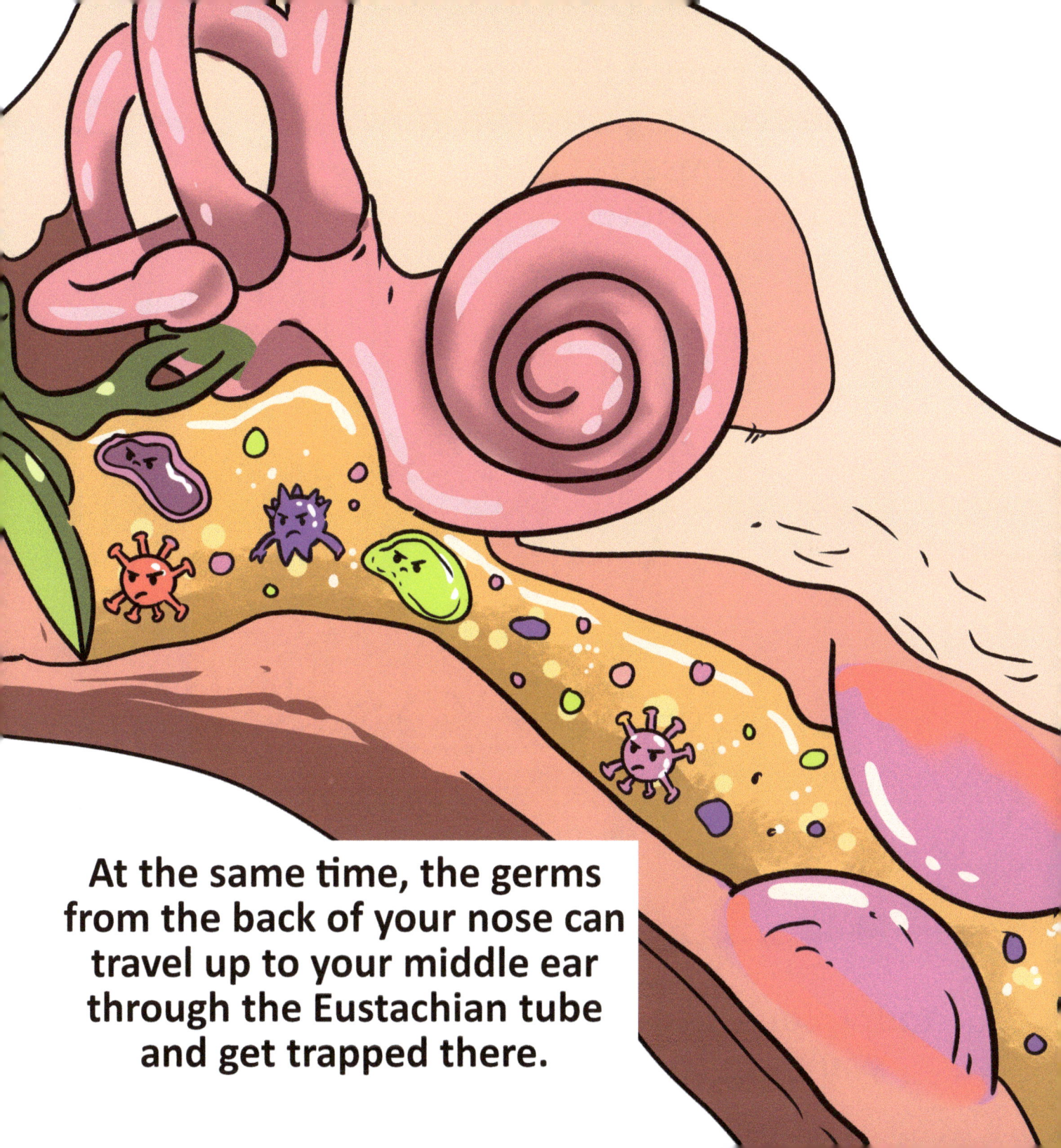

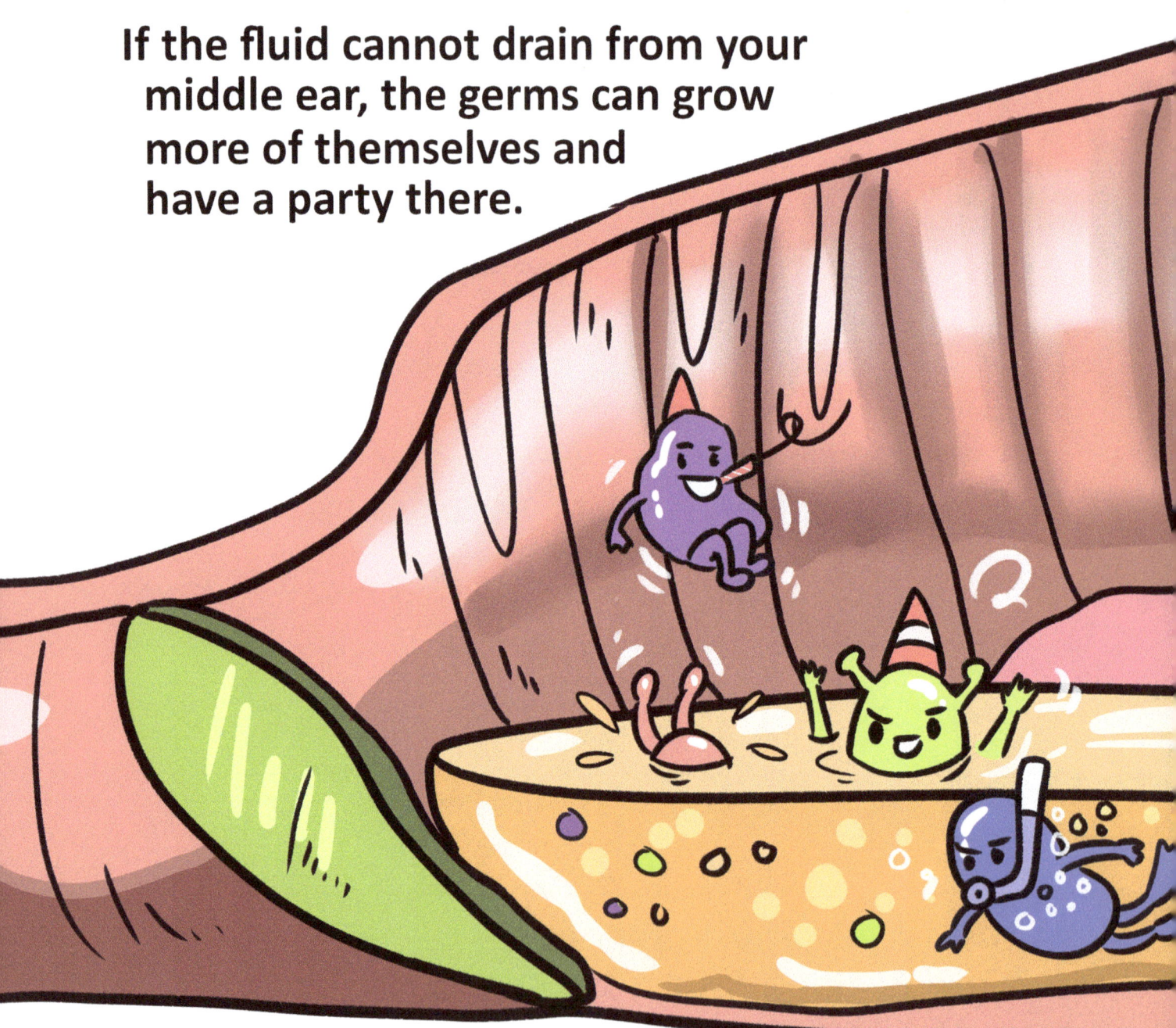

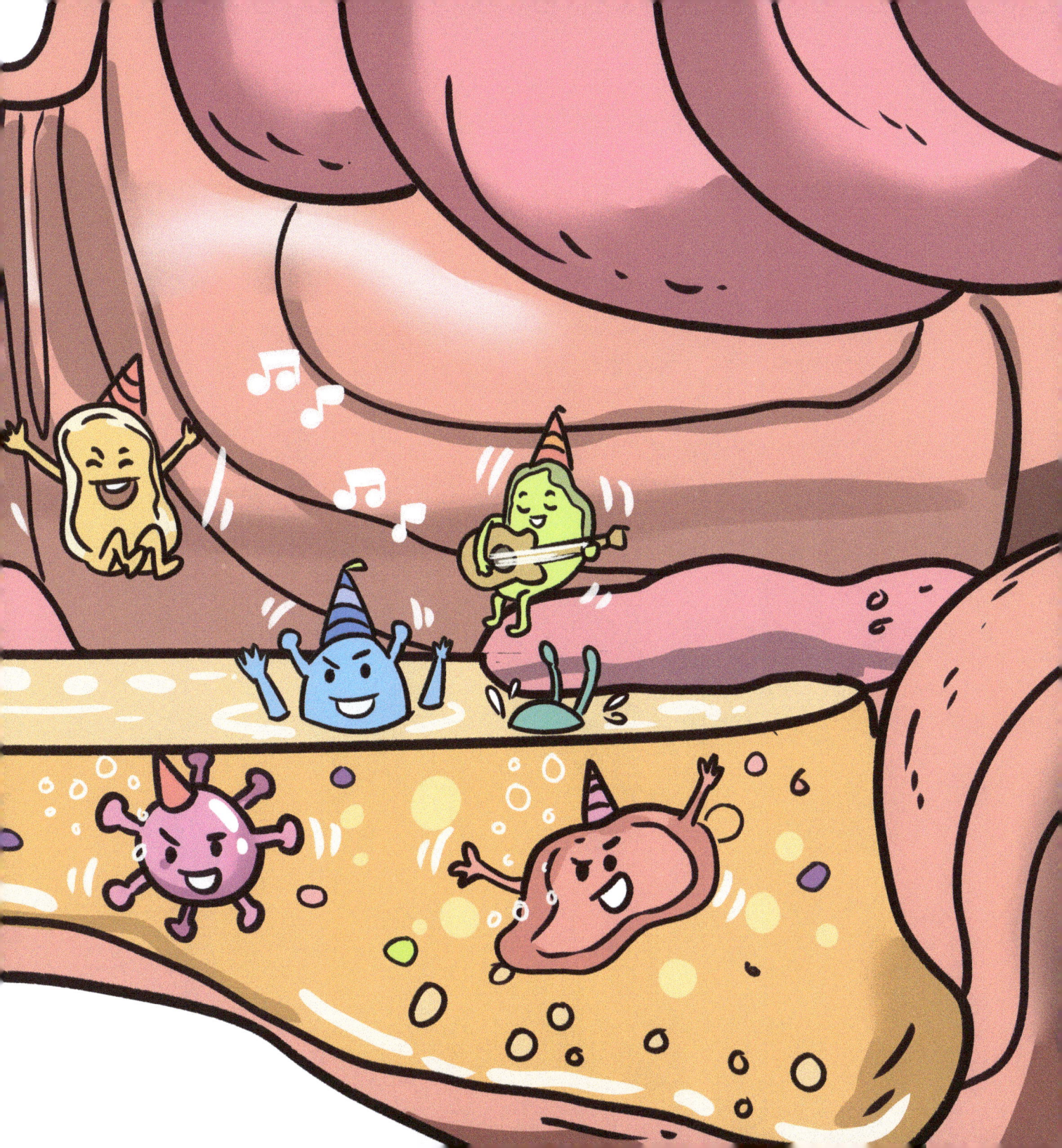

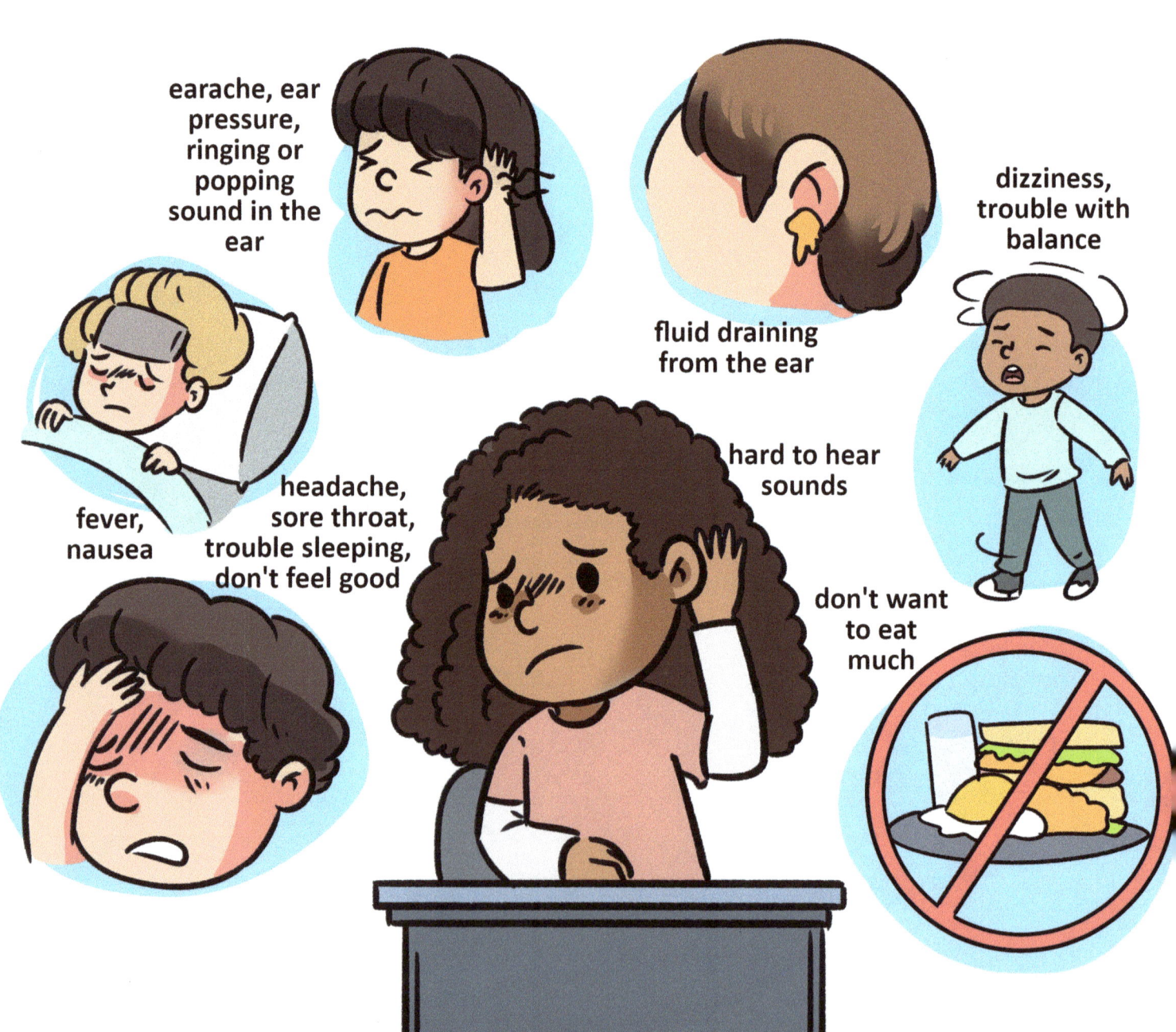

It's hard to learn new words or enjoy your favorite music if you cannot hear well.

Often, your ear infection improves by itself. If not, you may take medicine to get better.

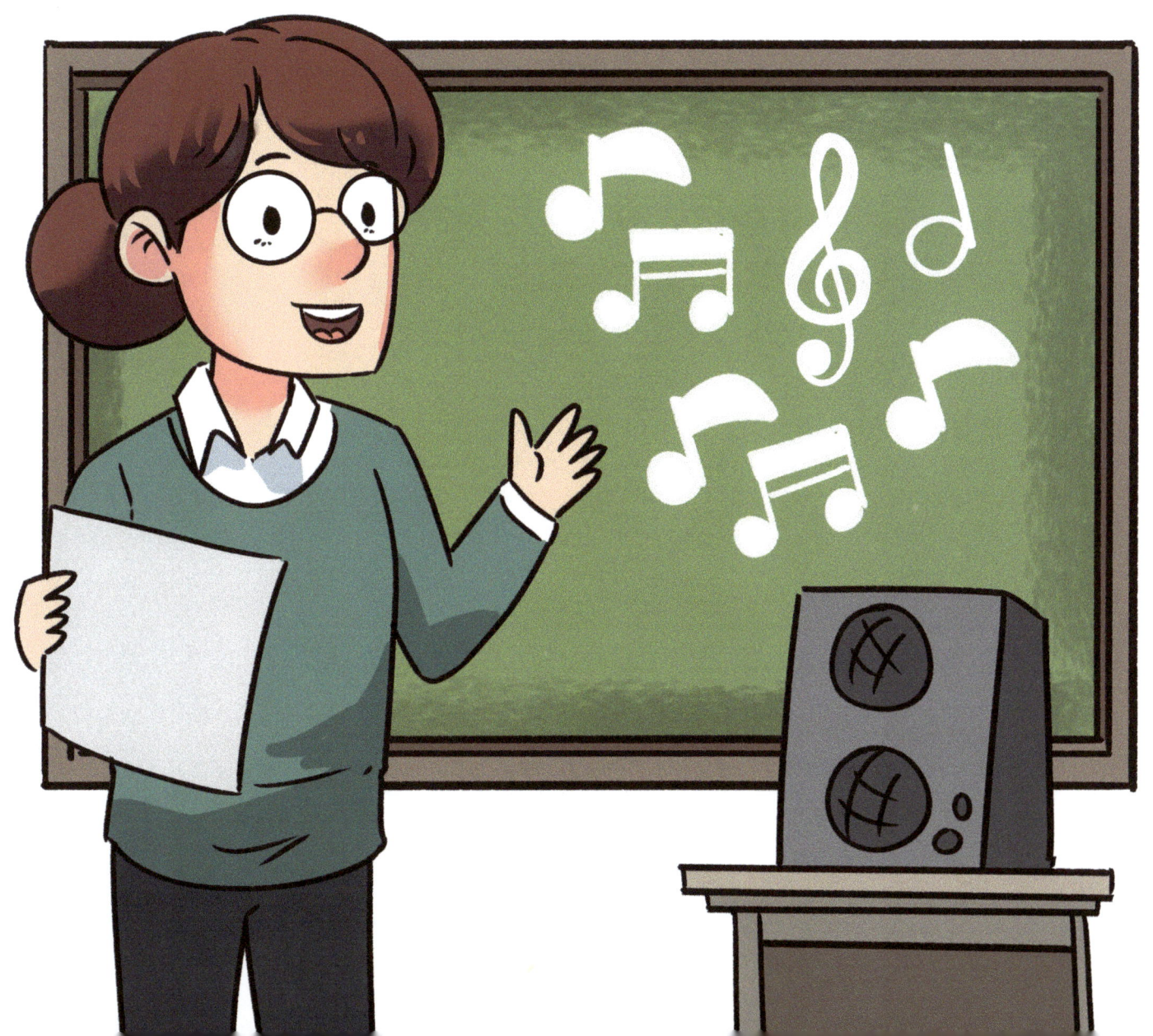

Your doctor, who is caring and gentle, can listen to your heart and lungs and check your nose and ears.

If you keep having middle ear infections, your doctor may recommend that you get an ear tube placed in your eardrum to help the fluid drain out to your ear canal.

Which ear did your doctor say you need an ear tube in?

Circle your answer below.

Left

Right

Both

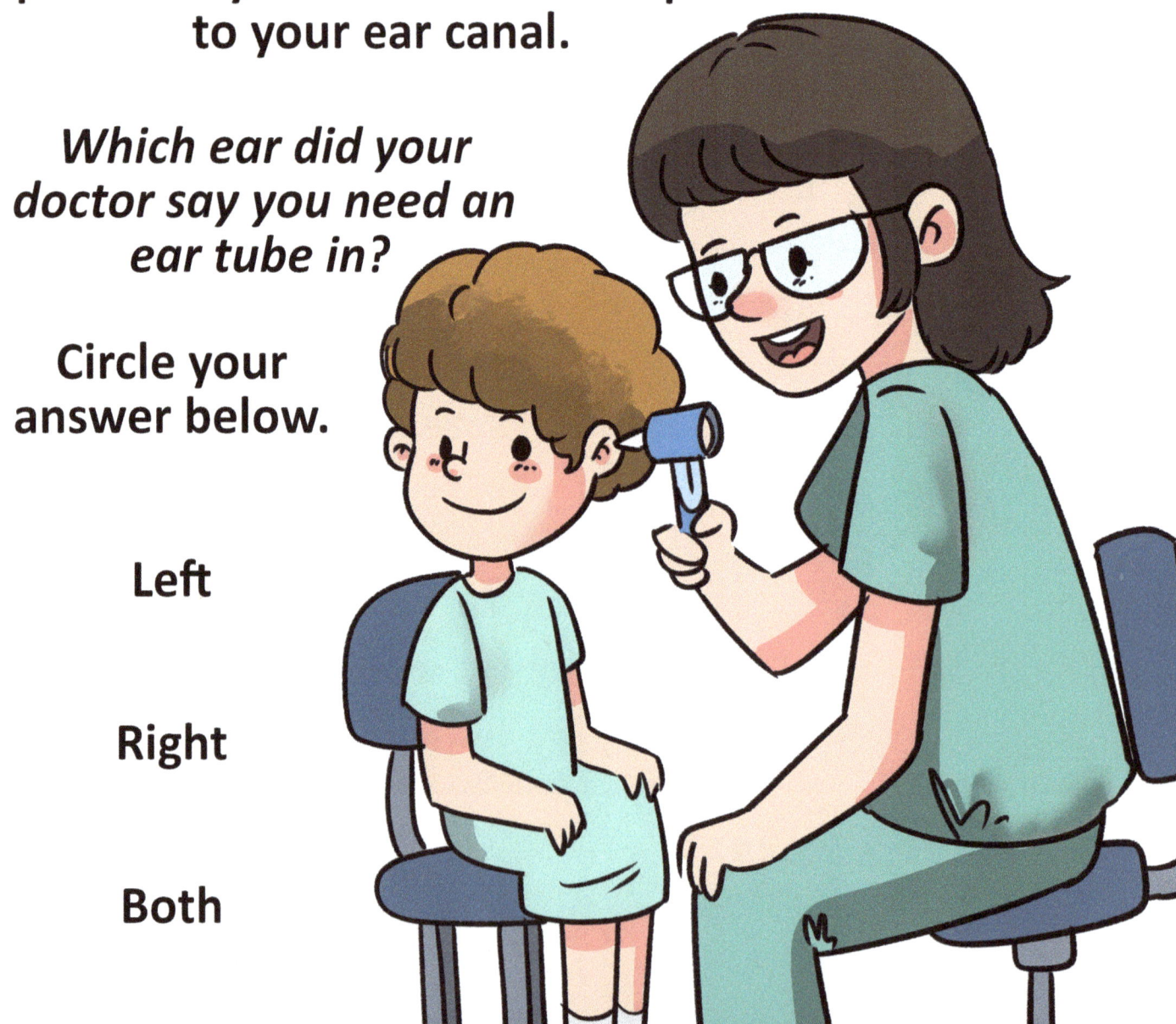

An ear tube is tiny and hollow and comes in different colors like white, blue, or green. It can be made of plastic or metal.

What color ear tube will you get? Circle yours below.

Blue   White   Green   Metal

Size of an American quarter dollar coin.

Size of ear tubes.

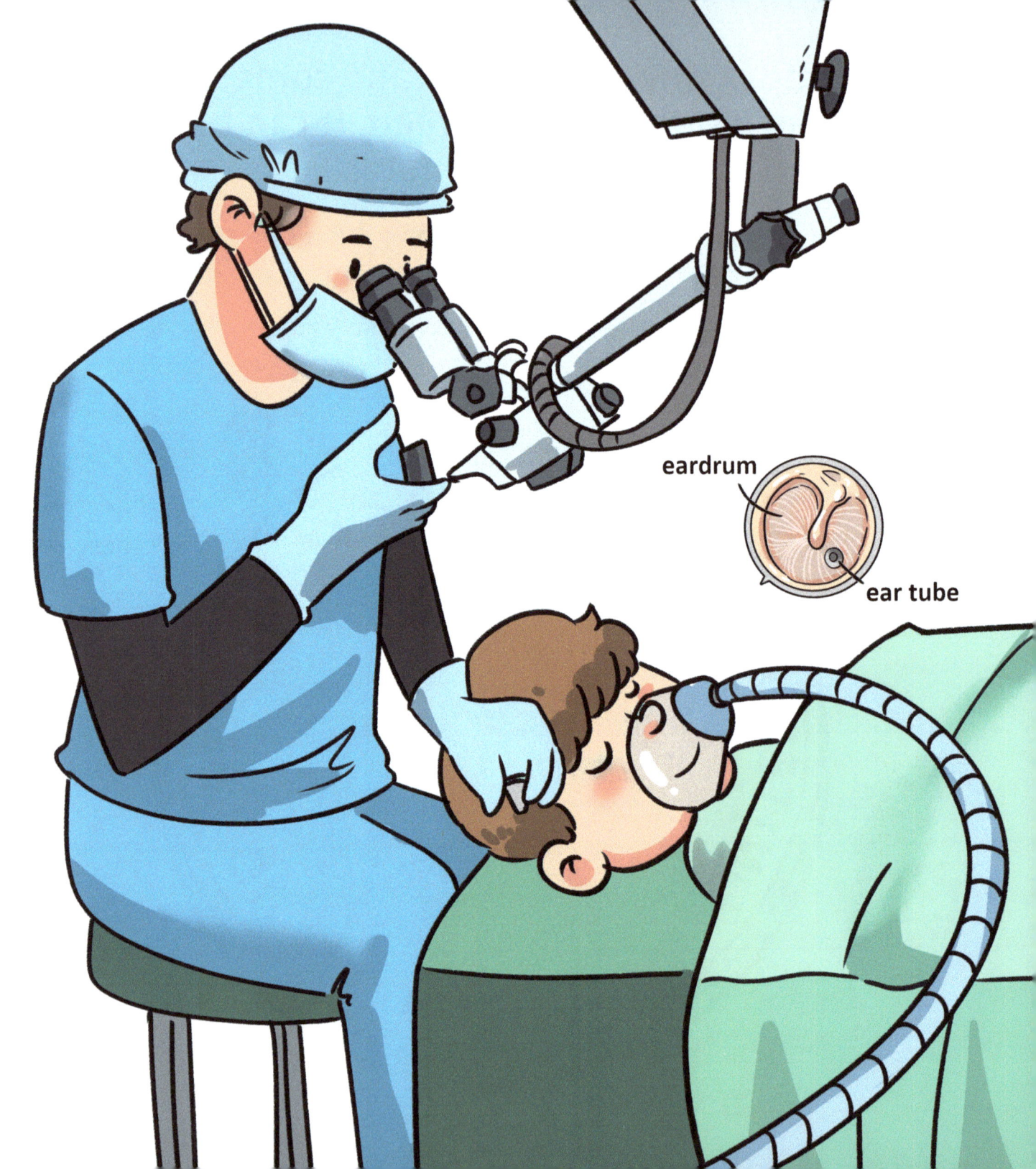

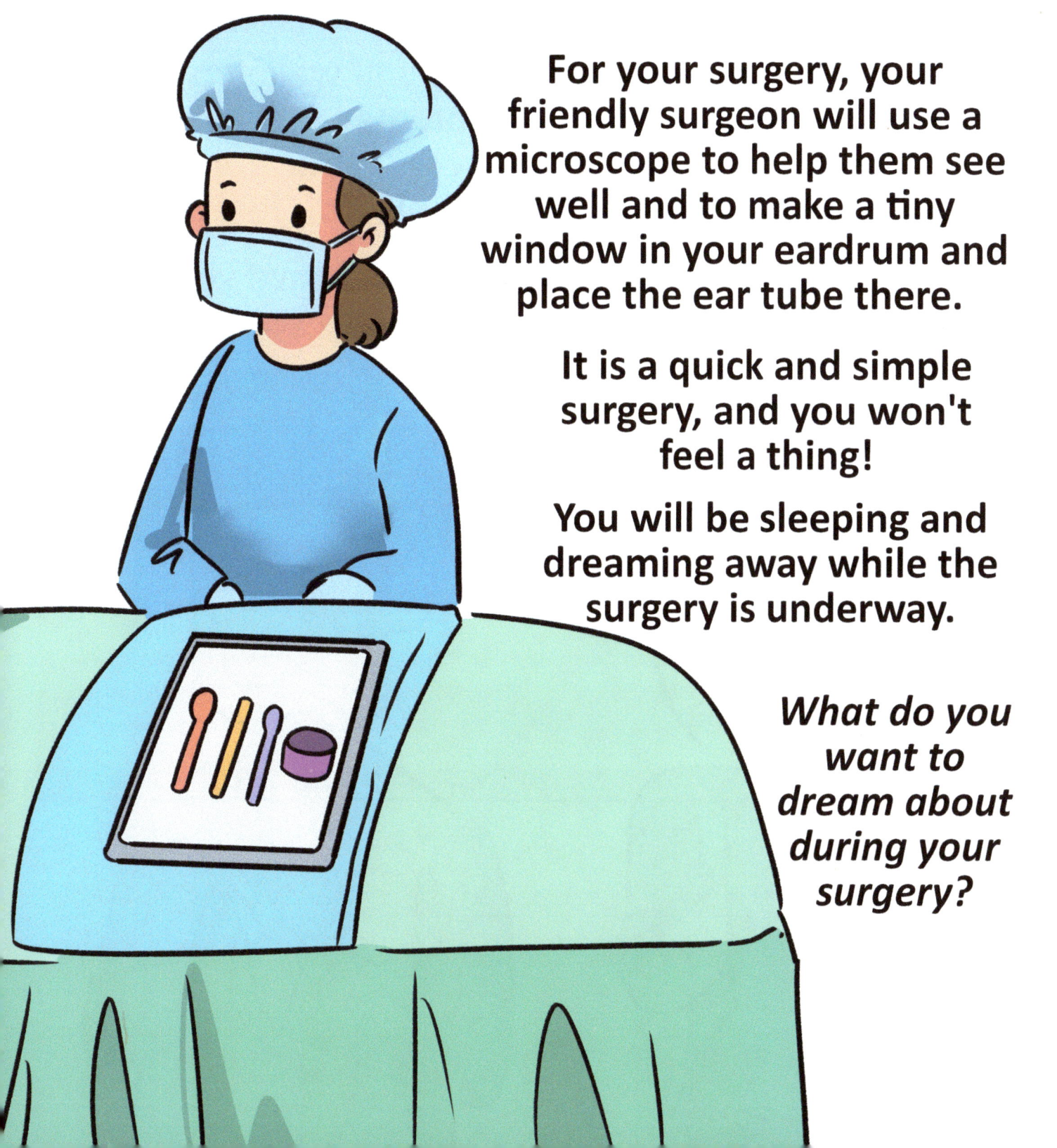

After your surgery is done, you will wake up in the hospital recovery room. You may feel a little uncomfortable, but don't worry; your nurse will give you special medicine to help you feel better.

Everyone in the room will see how brave you have been and will be so proud of you!

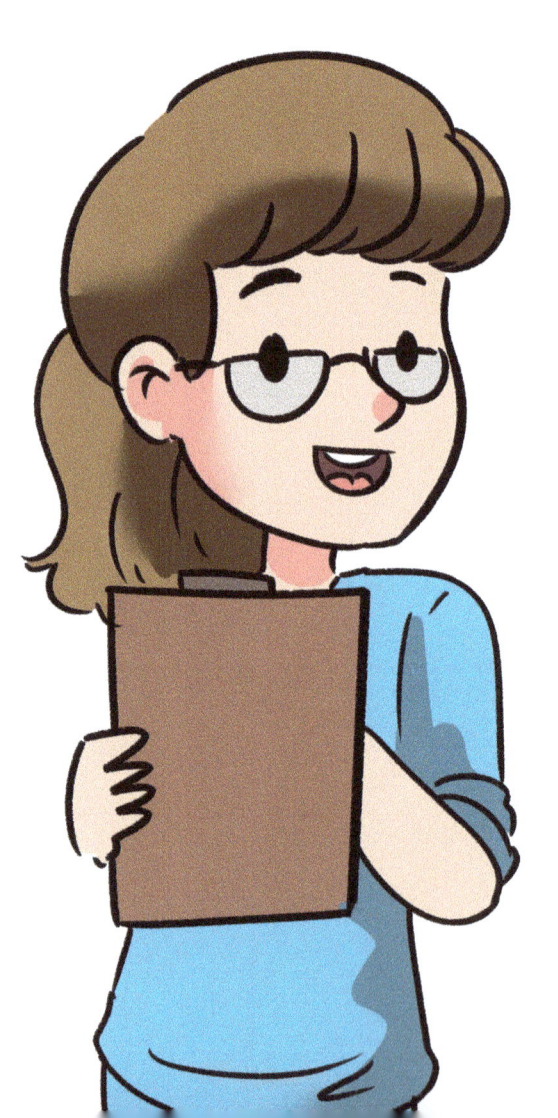
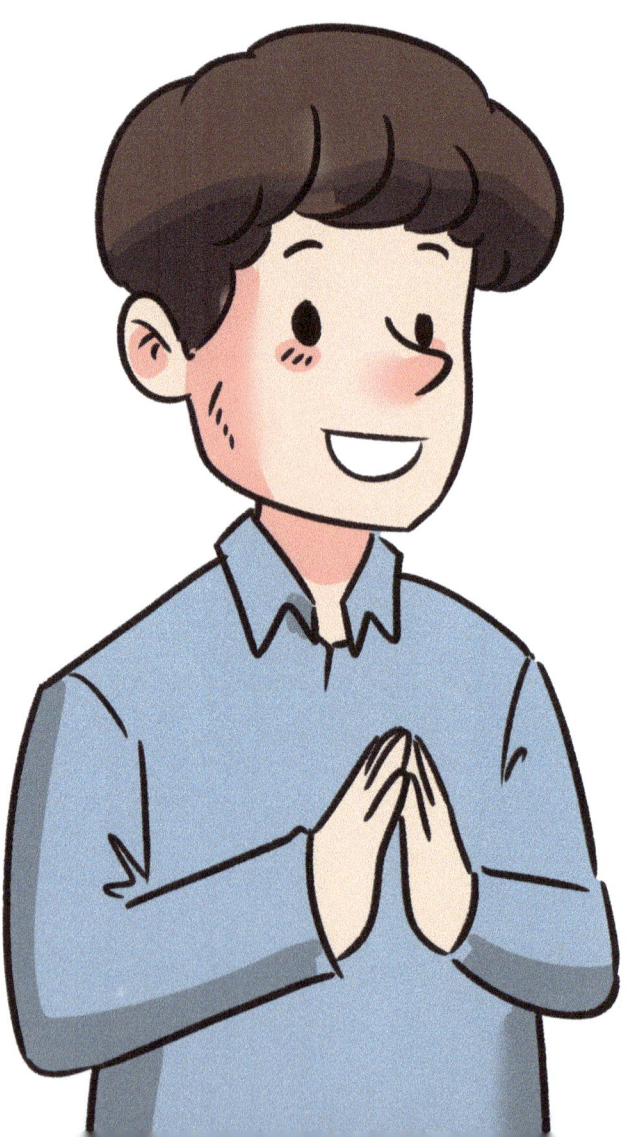

What are some things that will help you feel better and more comfortable after your surgery?

You are very brave,

_____!
(Write your name above)

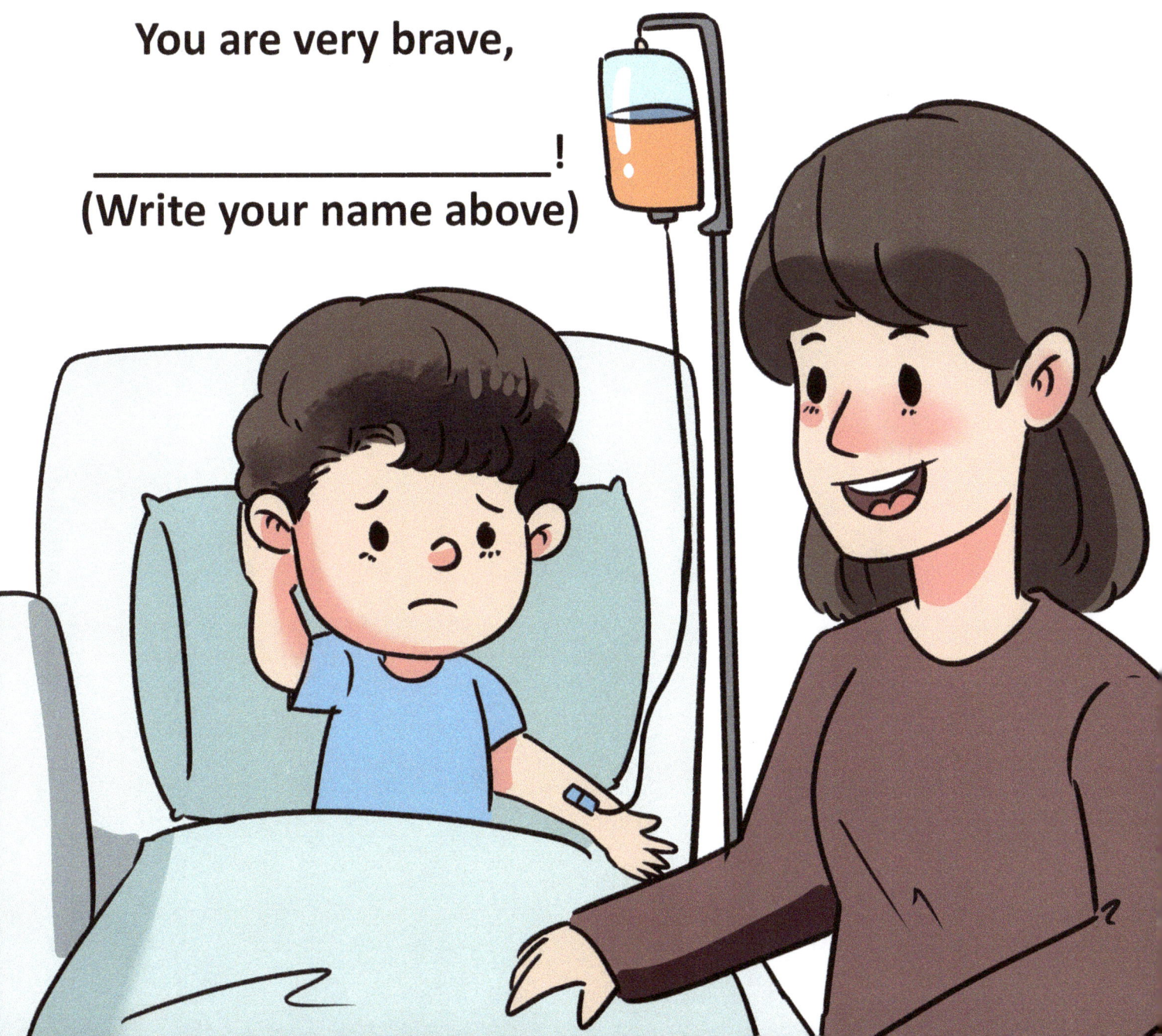

While you're recovering from your surgery, you may have a fever, may be a little sensitive to sounds, and may not feel like eating much.

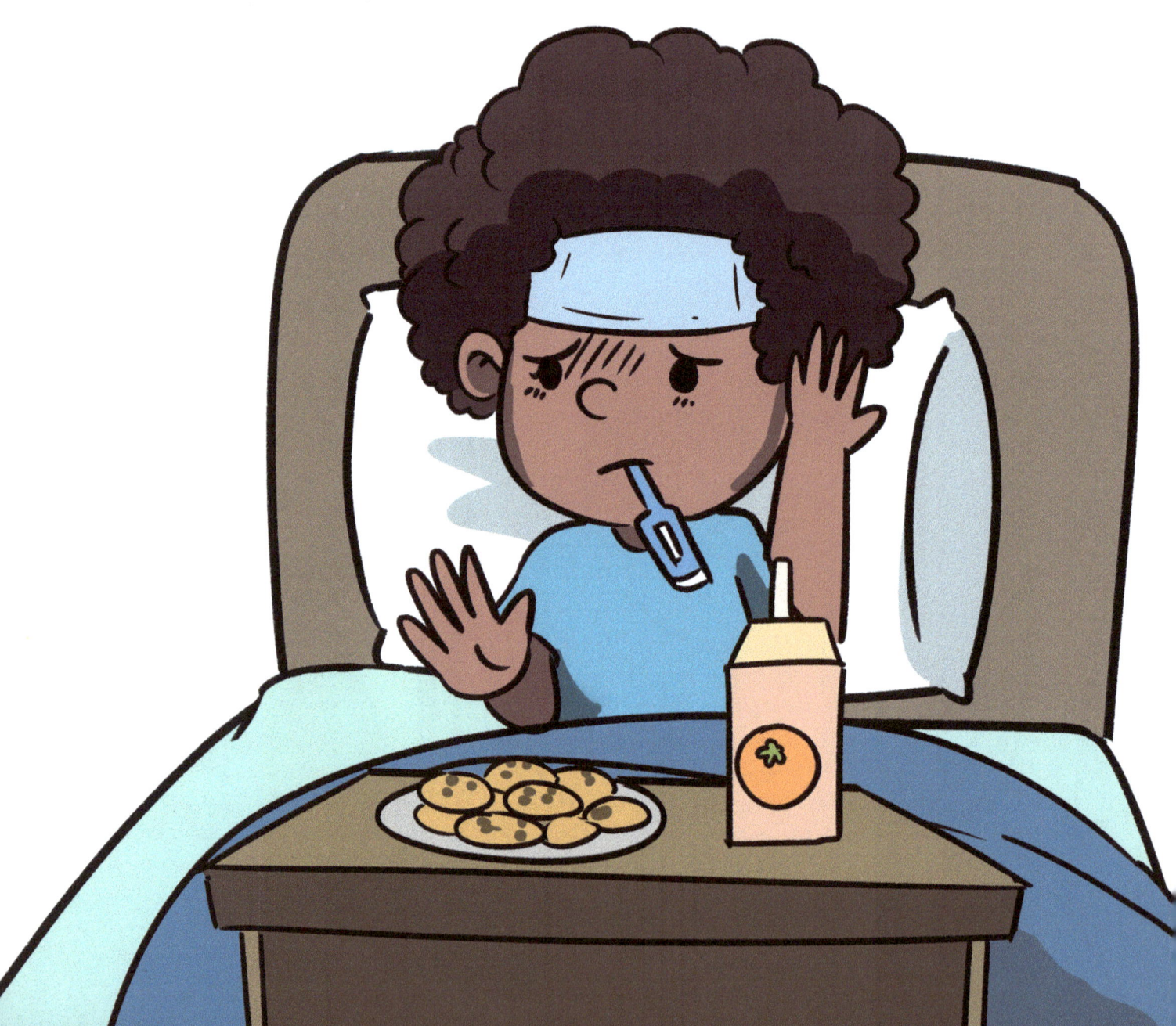

You may even feel some fluid come out of your ear. All of that is normal and will get better.

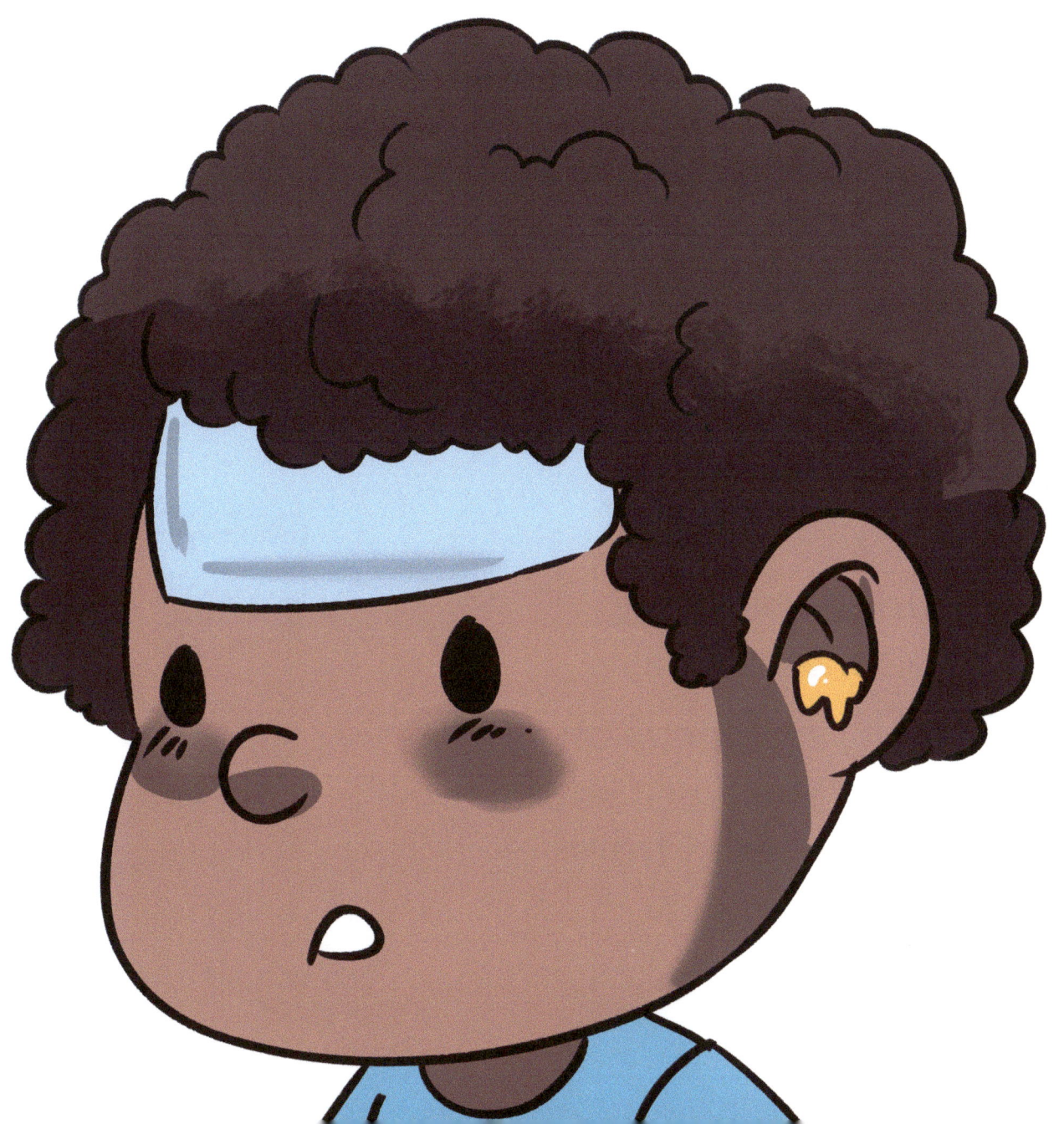

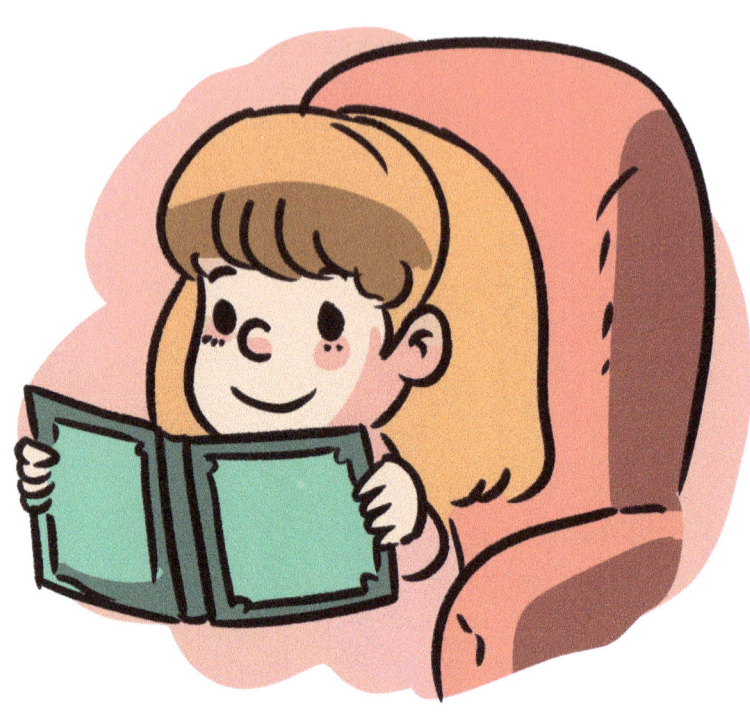

What are things you can do while you recover from your surgery?

During this time, please take it easy, *relax*, and focus on getting better until you have recovered from your surgery.

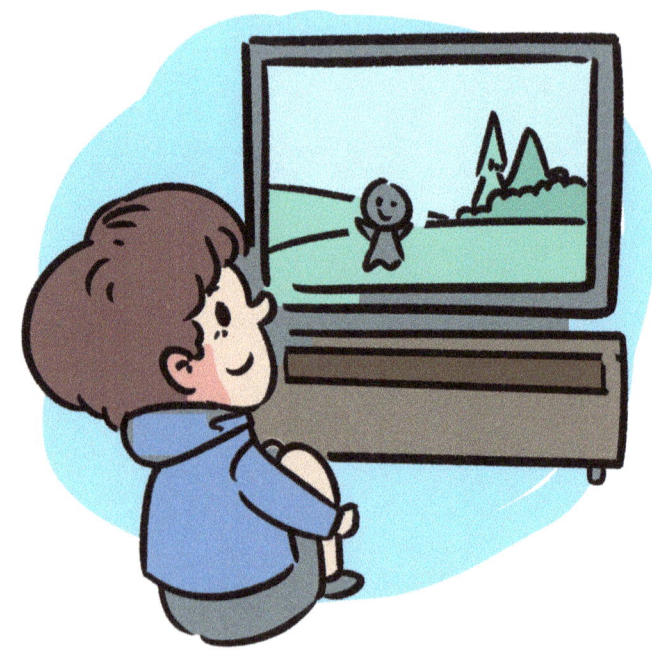

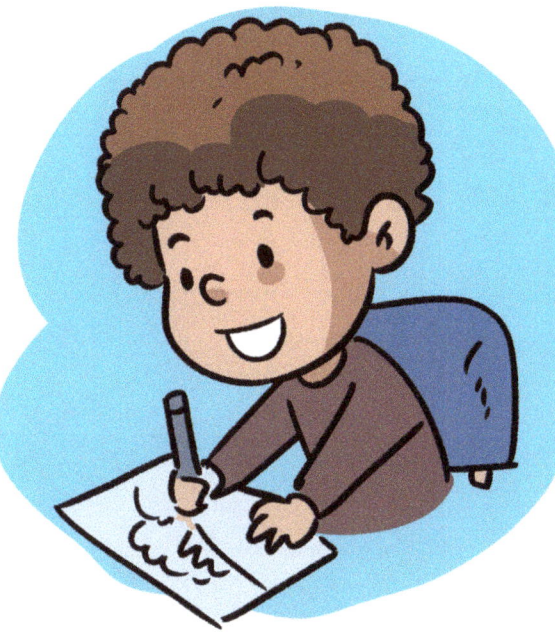

Once your ear tube is in place, any fluid in your middle ear can drain out easily, and you will feel and hear better.

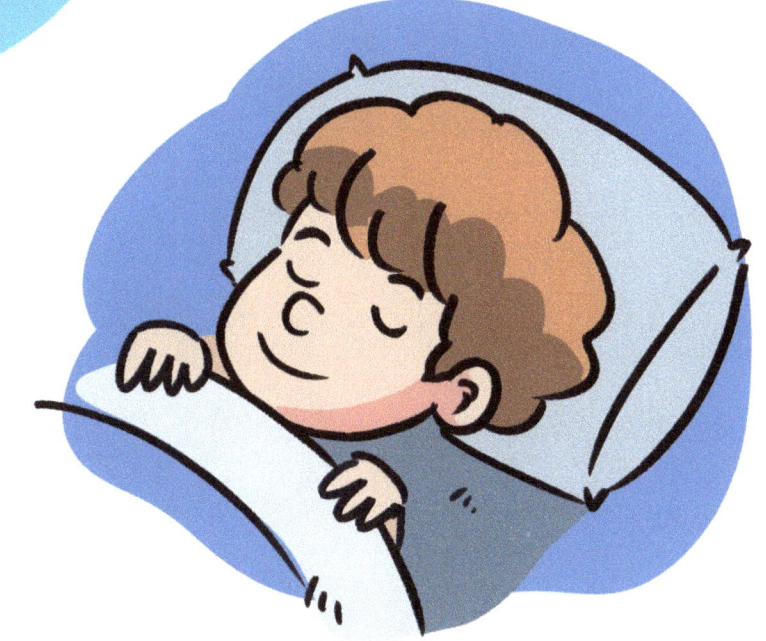

I plan to:

_____ Read books

_____ Watch movies

_____ Draw or color

_____ Rest

Other: _____

You will probably get special drops for your ear. The drops may feel a little cold but they help fight off the germs to help you feel better faster.

Don't worry; your parent or guardian will help you.

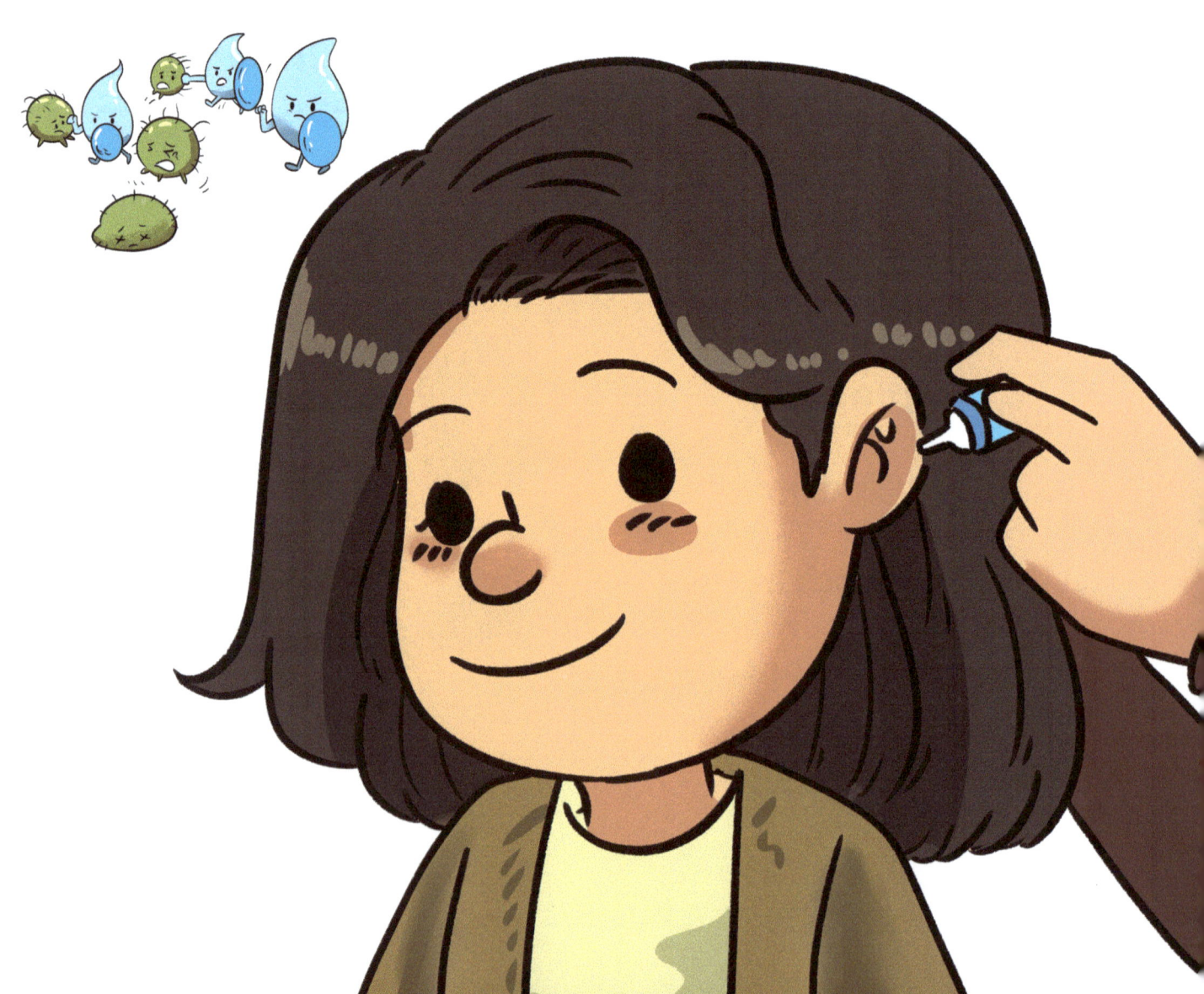

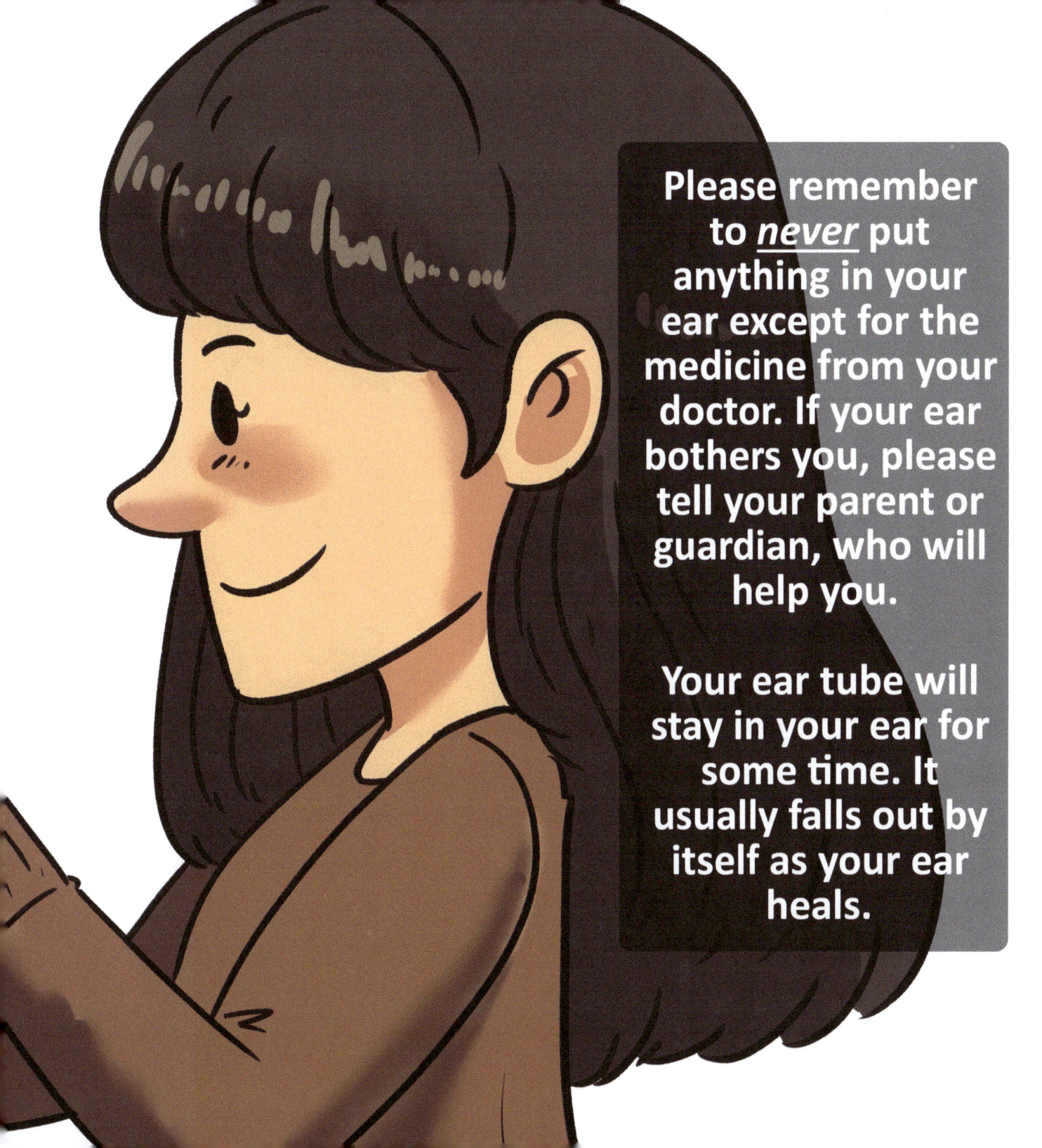

If you keep your head out of the water, you can bathe or even swim in clean water without earplugs.

But if you prefer to use earplugs, you absolutely can.

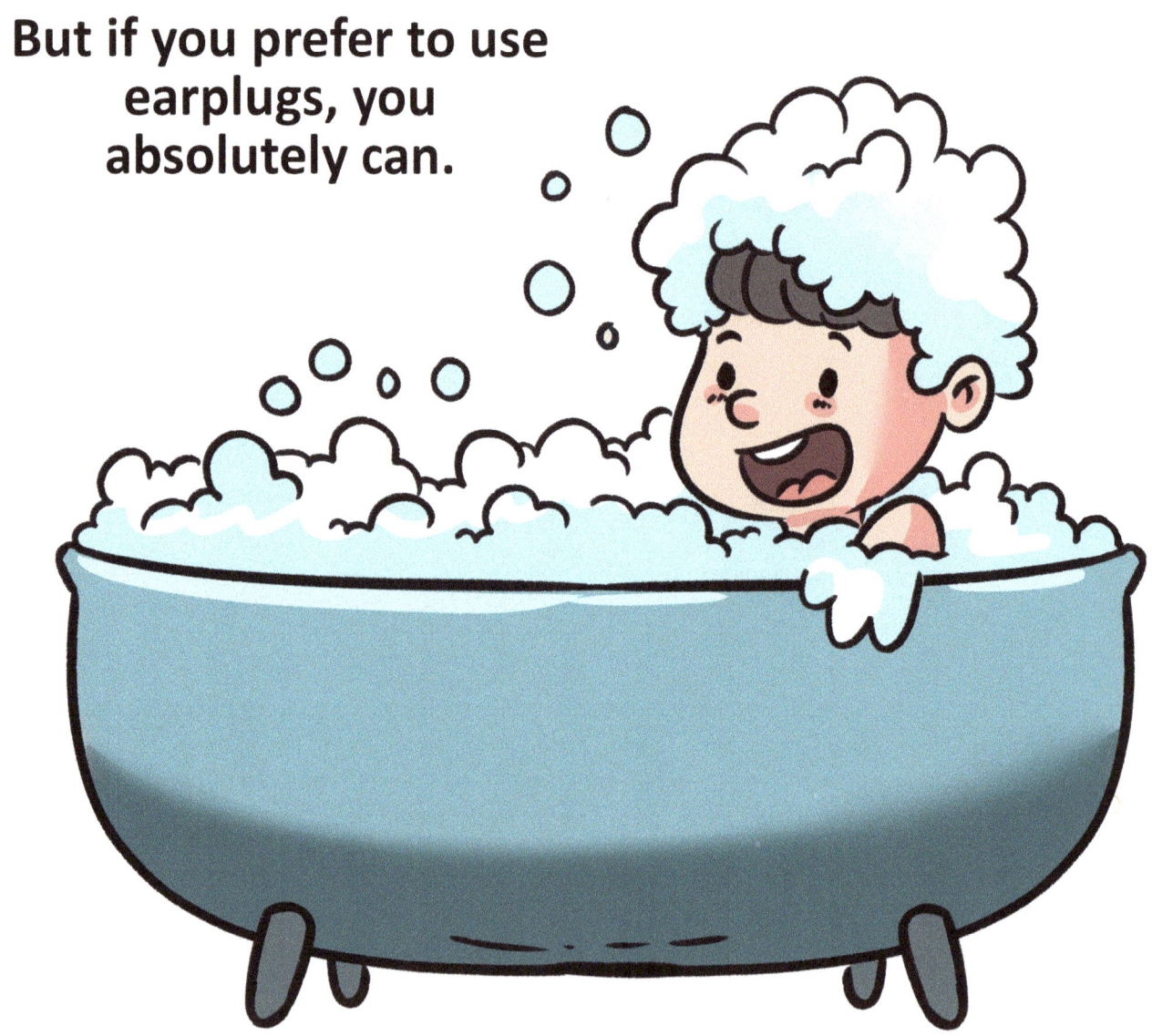

Don't worry; your doctor will tell your parent or guardian how to take care of your ear while it's healing.

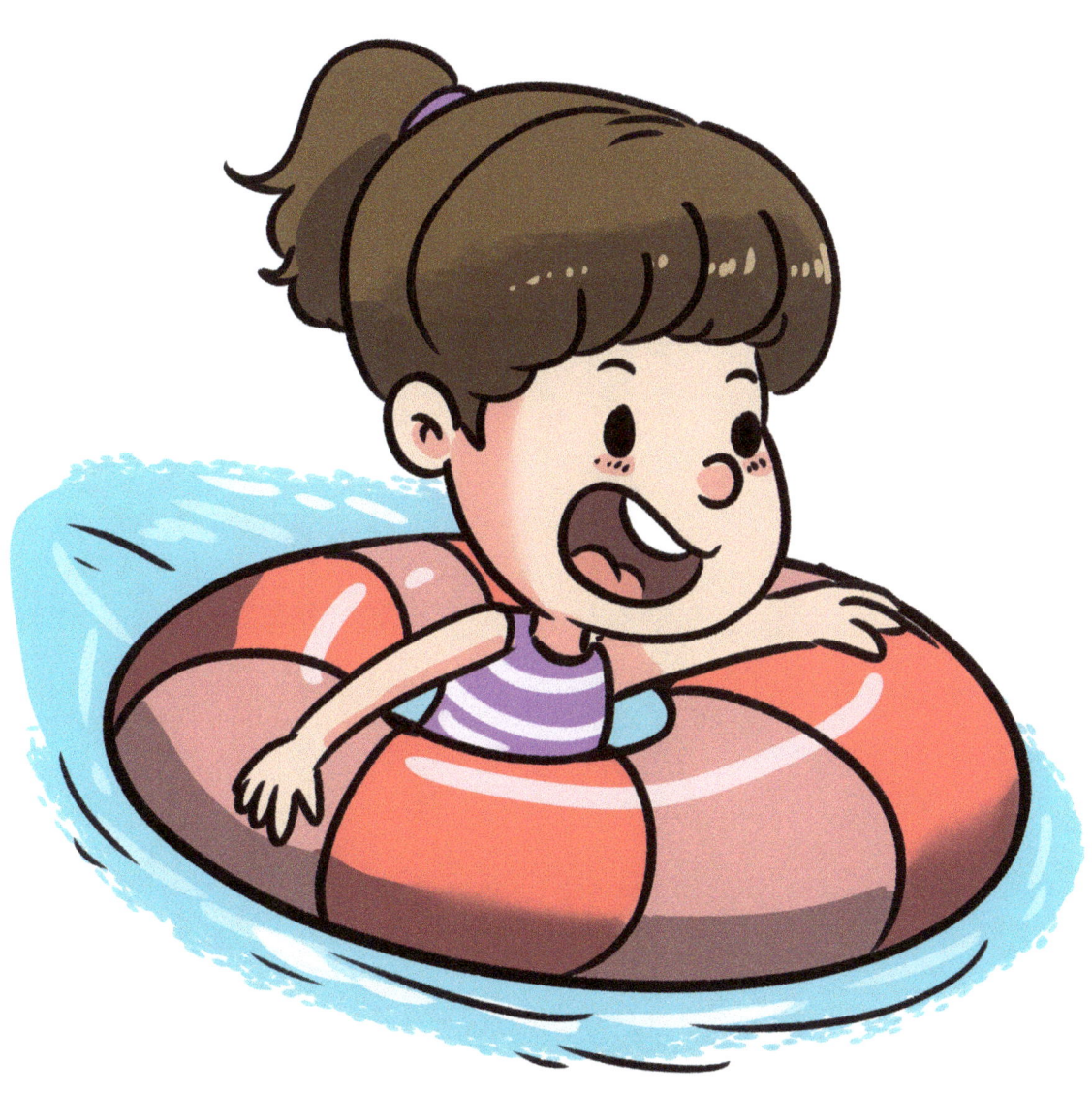

As long as you have your ear tube, you will see your doctor occasionally to make sure it's working and that your ear is healing well.

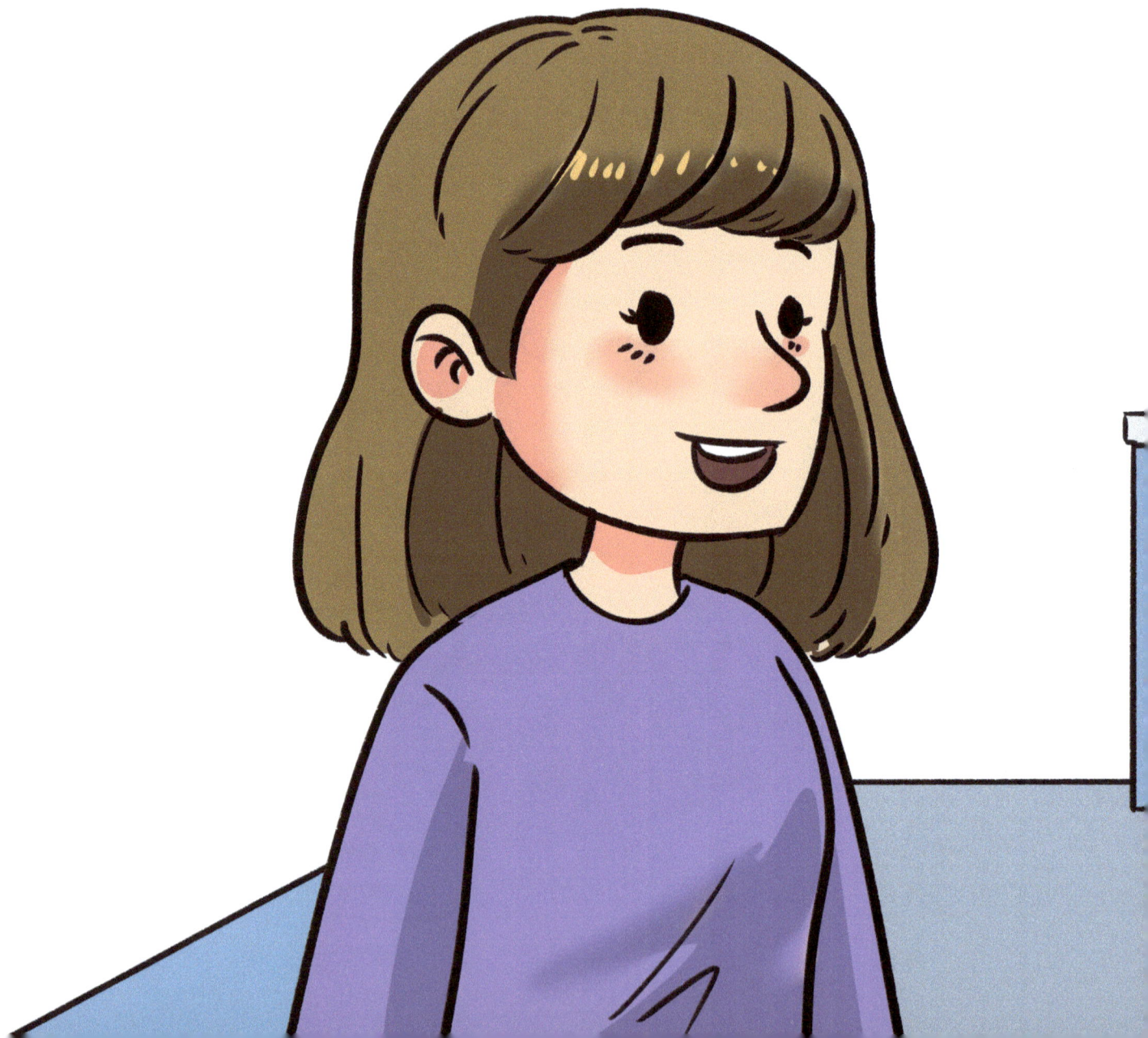

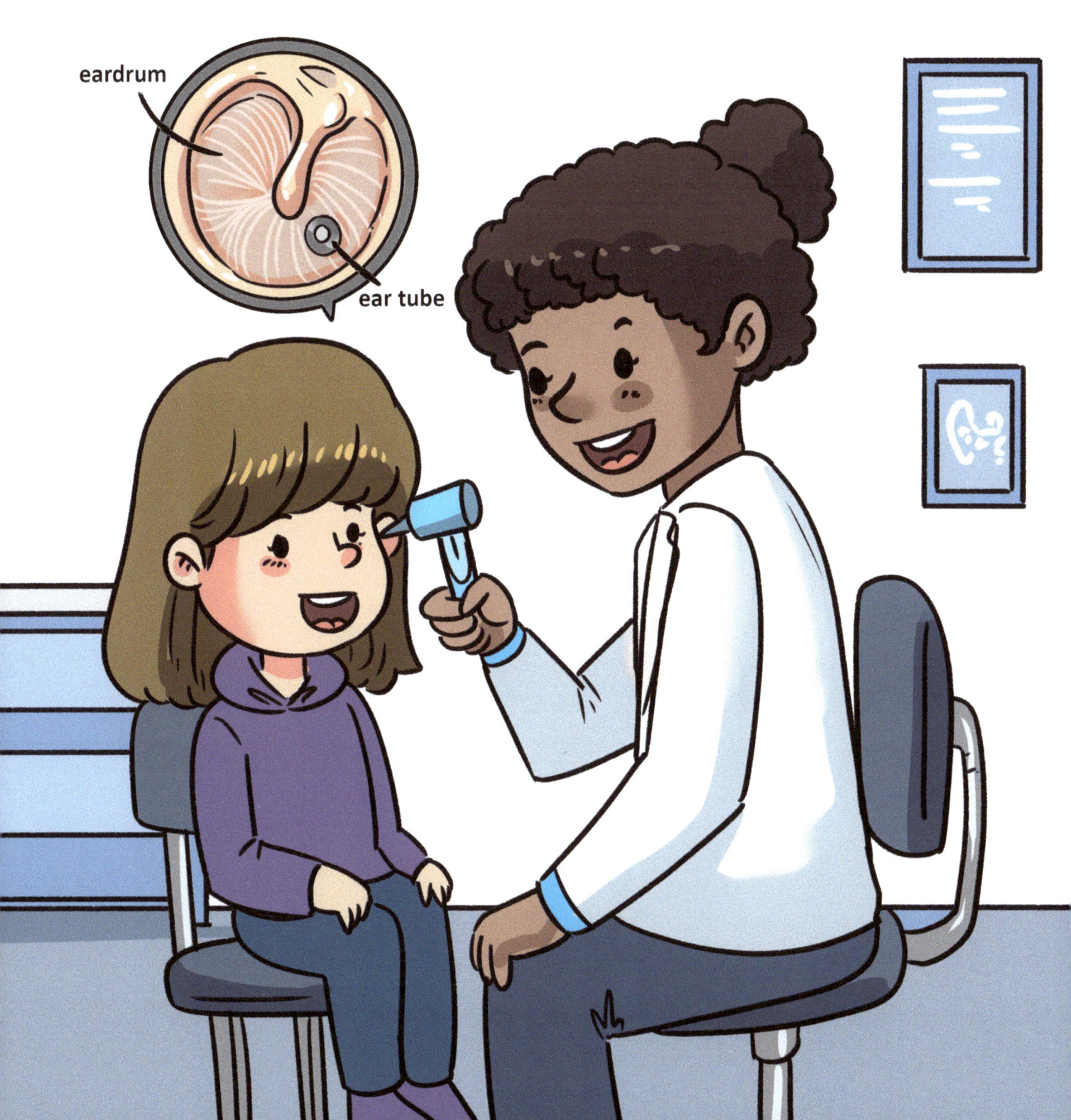

What will you do after you get your ear tube(s)?

A party? A celebration?

What's your favorite way to celebrate?

Draw or write your party plan below.

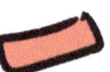

Speedy recovery!

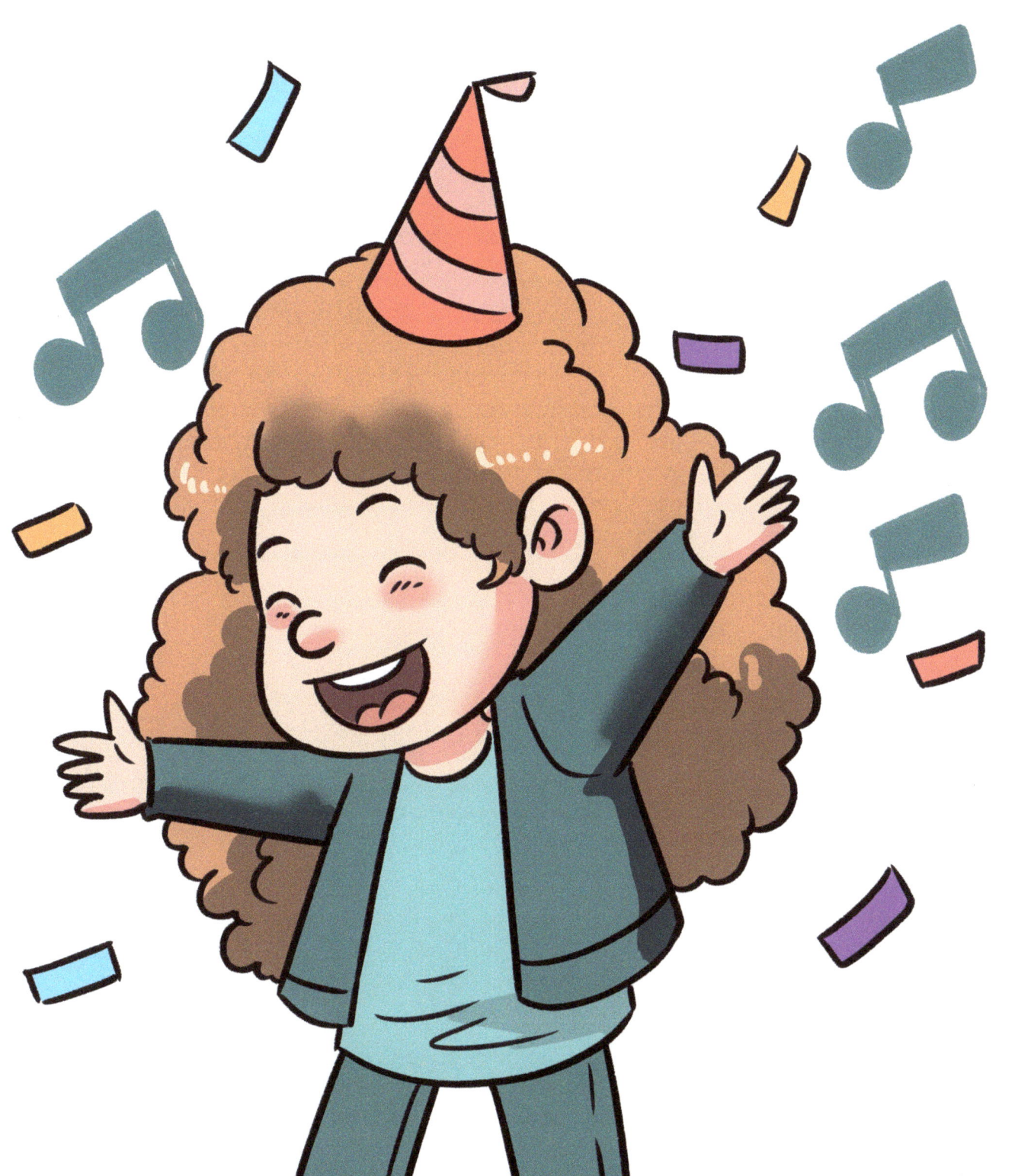

Notes for Parent/Guardian

• Placement of the intravenous (IV) catheter in this young age group is typically done *after* your child is asleep in the operating room. In some cases, the IV catheter may not be necessary.

• After the surgery, it is common for children to feel confused, disoriented, or irritable, and they may cry, sob, kick, scream, or thrash around. It normally takes about one hour for the anesthesia to wear off.

• Post-surgery instructions/restrictions:
Your child's doctor should give you specific instructions on (1) what your child can and cannot do during the recovery period, (2) the duration of the post-surgical restrictions, and (3) any post-surgical follow-ups. Additionally, (4) they should instruct what to watch out for and when it is necessary for you to bring your child back to the hospital in case of an emergency. If they forget, please kindly remind them and obtain these instructions/restrictions before leaving the hospital.

Disclaimer

Please note that the illustrations are not drawn to scale.

This book is written for informational, educational, and personal growth purposes and should not be used as a substitute for medical advice.

Please consult your child's doctor if they need medical attention and to ensure the information in this book pertains to your child's medical condition and needs. I cannot guarantee what your child experiences is exactly what is being discussed in this book.

The author and the publisher are not responsible, either directly or indirectly, for any damages, monetary losses, or reparations due to information in this book. By reading this book, the readers agree not to hold the author and the publisher responsible for any losses as a result of any errors, inaccuracies, or omissions in this book.

Please keep in mind that your child's experience depends on the location, the facility, their medical condition, and the healthcare team. Please use this book in conjunction with your child's doctor's advice. Thank you.

Did this picture book help your child in some way?
If so, I would love to hear about it!

www.amazon.com/gp/product-review/B0DTV85K79

For other book titles, please visit:

www.fzwbooks.com

Connect with the author

email: books@fzwbooks.com
facebook/instagram: @FZWbooks

About the Author

Dr. Fei Zheng-Ward is a clinical anesthesiologist who understands the apprehension patients (both adults and children) may have surrounding their upcoming surgery. Her goal in her medical books is to bring useful information to patients so they have a better understanding and appreciation of what happens leading up to, during, and after surgery. She wants readers to be more empowered to make informed decisions and to feel more at ease with their surgery.

As a practicing physician, she takes pride in being respected for her attention to detail, commitment to providing compassionate and personalized patient care, and strong presence in patient advocacy in the perioperative period for each of her patients. She understands the importance of physical and emotional well-being and advocates for patient autonomy.

Her other children's books aim to bring laughter into your home, encourage children to be more helpful at home, and inspire a love of reading.

She is an award-winning author for her book titled ***What to Expect and How to Prepare for Your Surgery***.

More about Dr. Fei Zheng-Ward:

* Board Certified Anesthesiologist

* Anesthesiology Residency Training at The Johns Hopkins Hospital in Baltimore, MD

* Master in Public Health (MPH) degree from Dartmouth Medical School in Hanover, NH

Books by the author

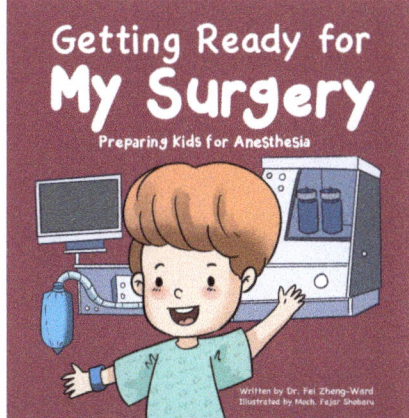
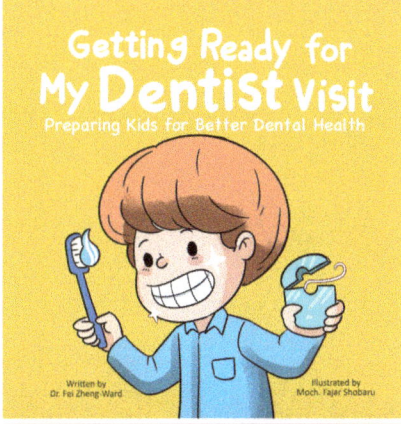
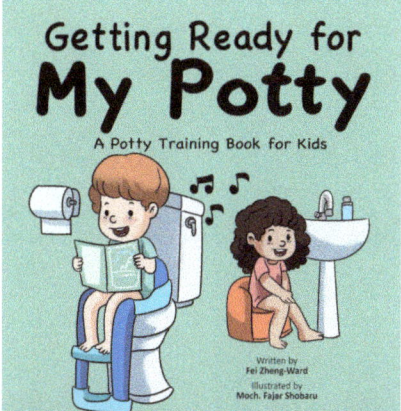
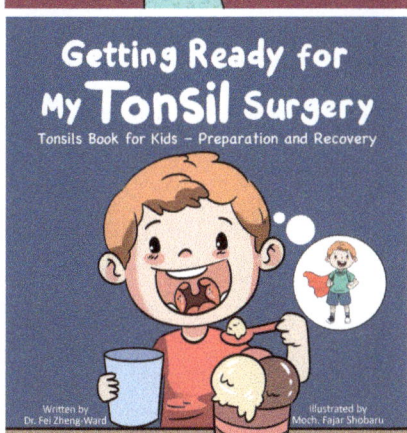
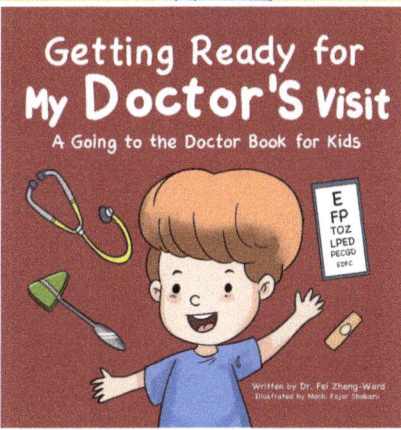
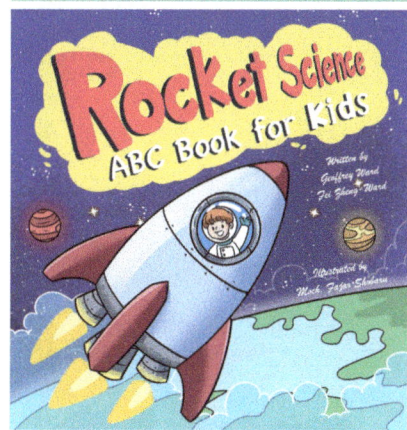
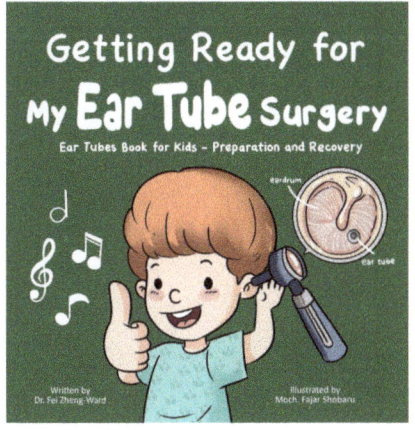
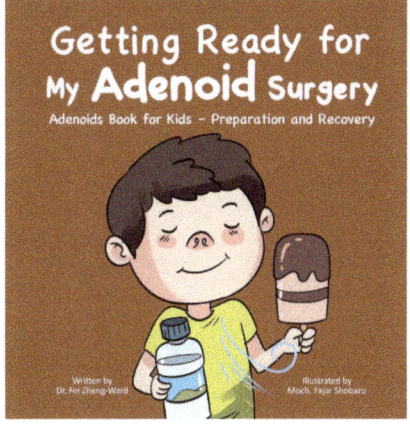
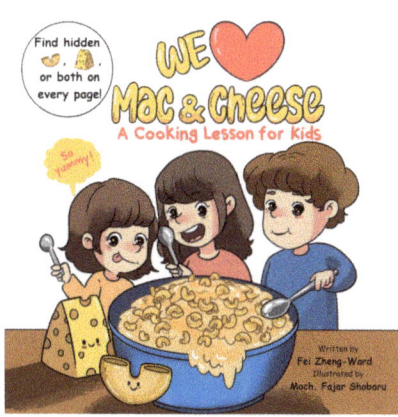

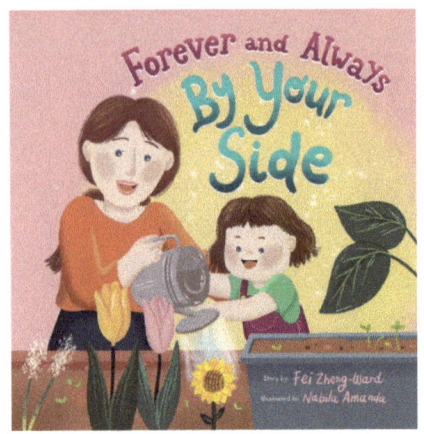
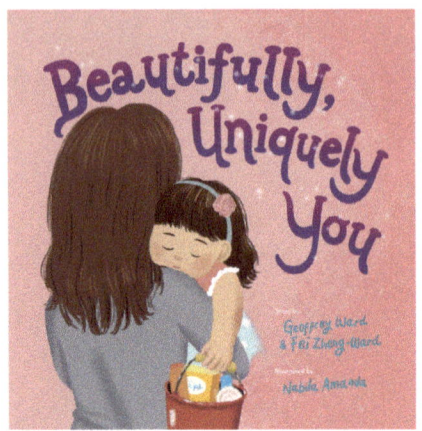
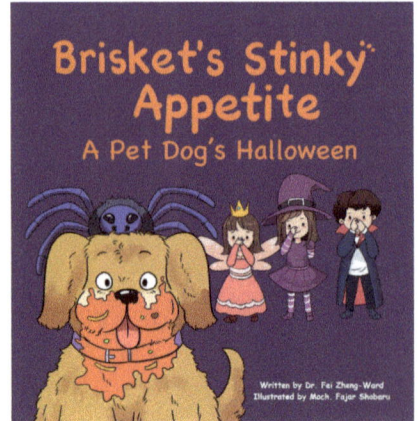
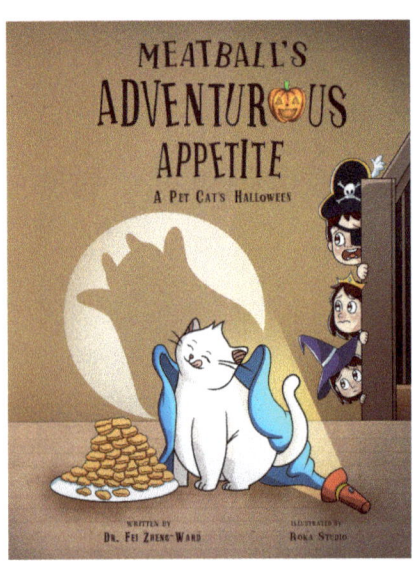
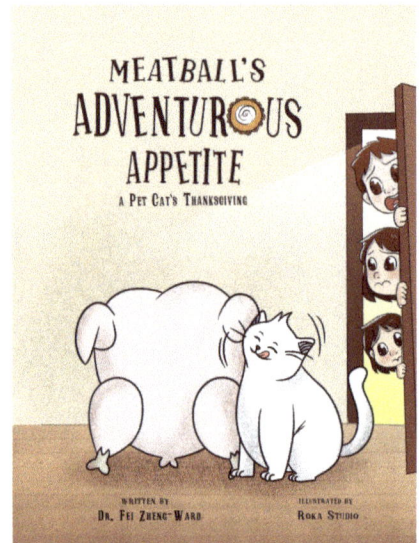
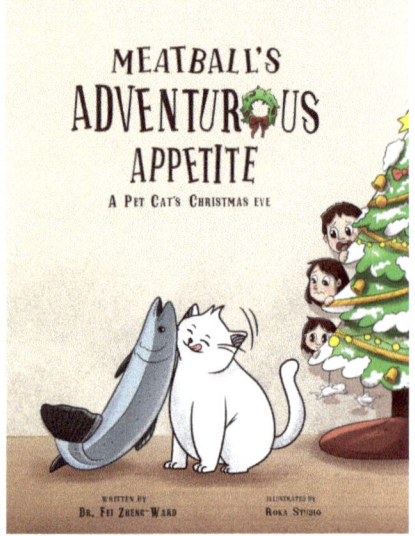
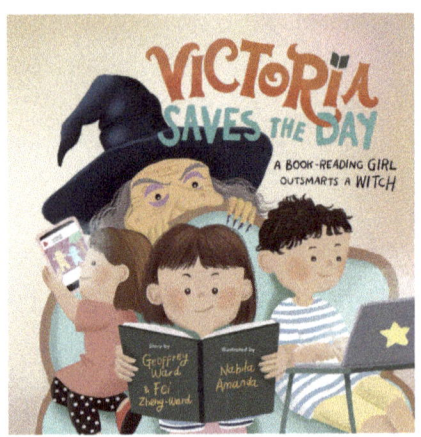
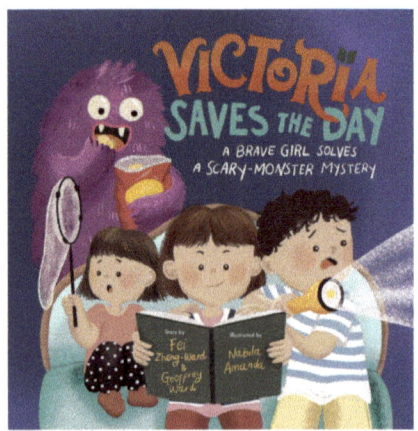
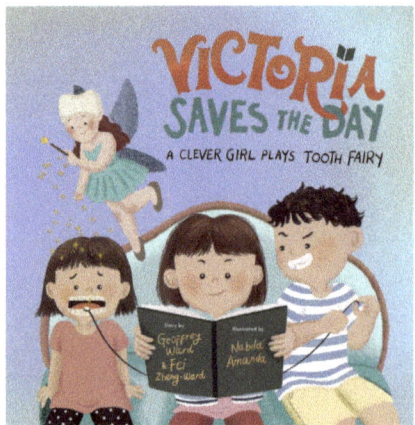

www.ingramcontent.com/pod-product-compliance
Lightning Source LLC
Chambersburg PA
CBHW040001040426
42337CB00032B/5177